CAT
BREEDS

A Picture Book for People Who Like Cats, Not Words

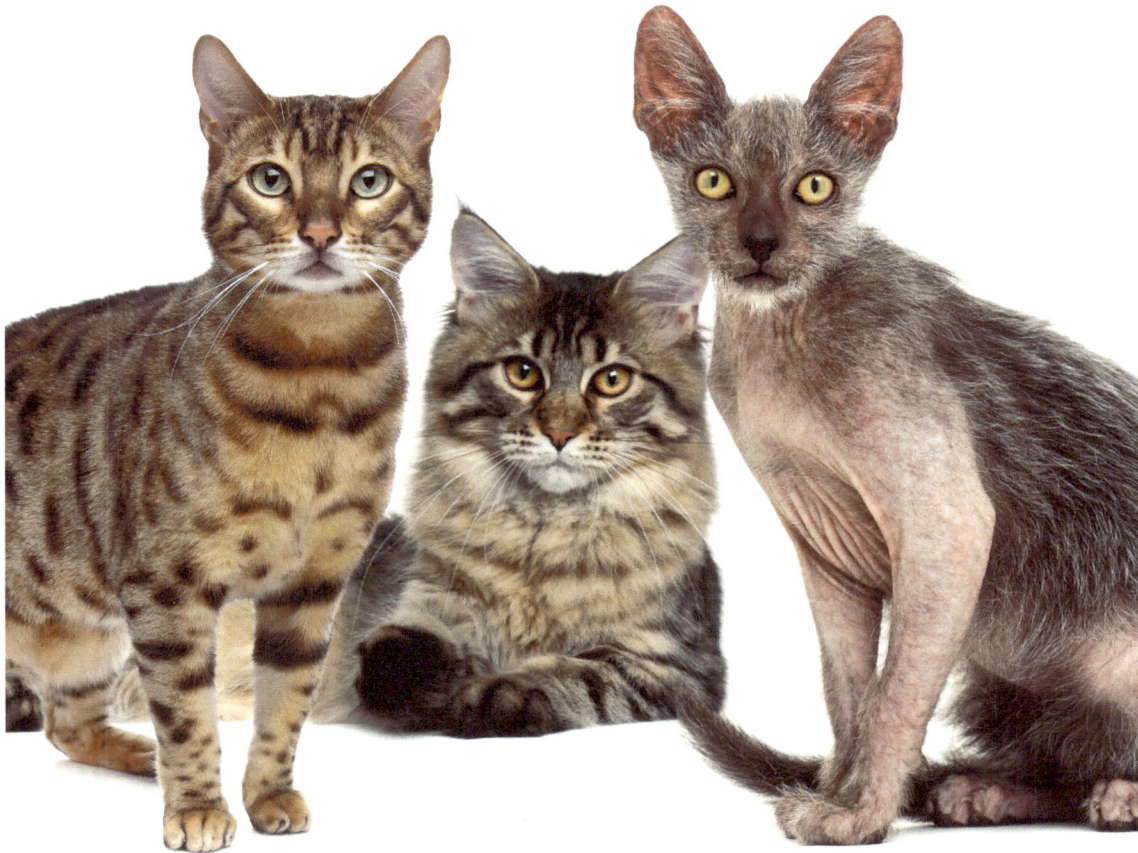

Copyright © 2020 by Lasting Happiness
ISBN: 978-1-9995487-9-7

American Curl

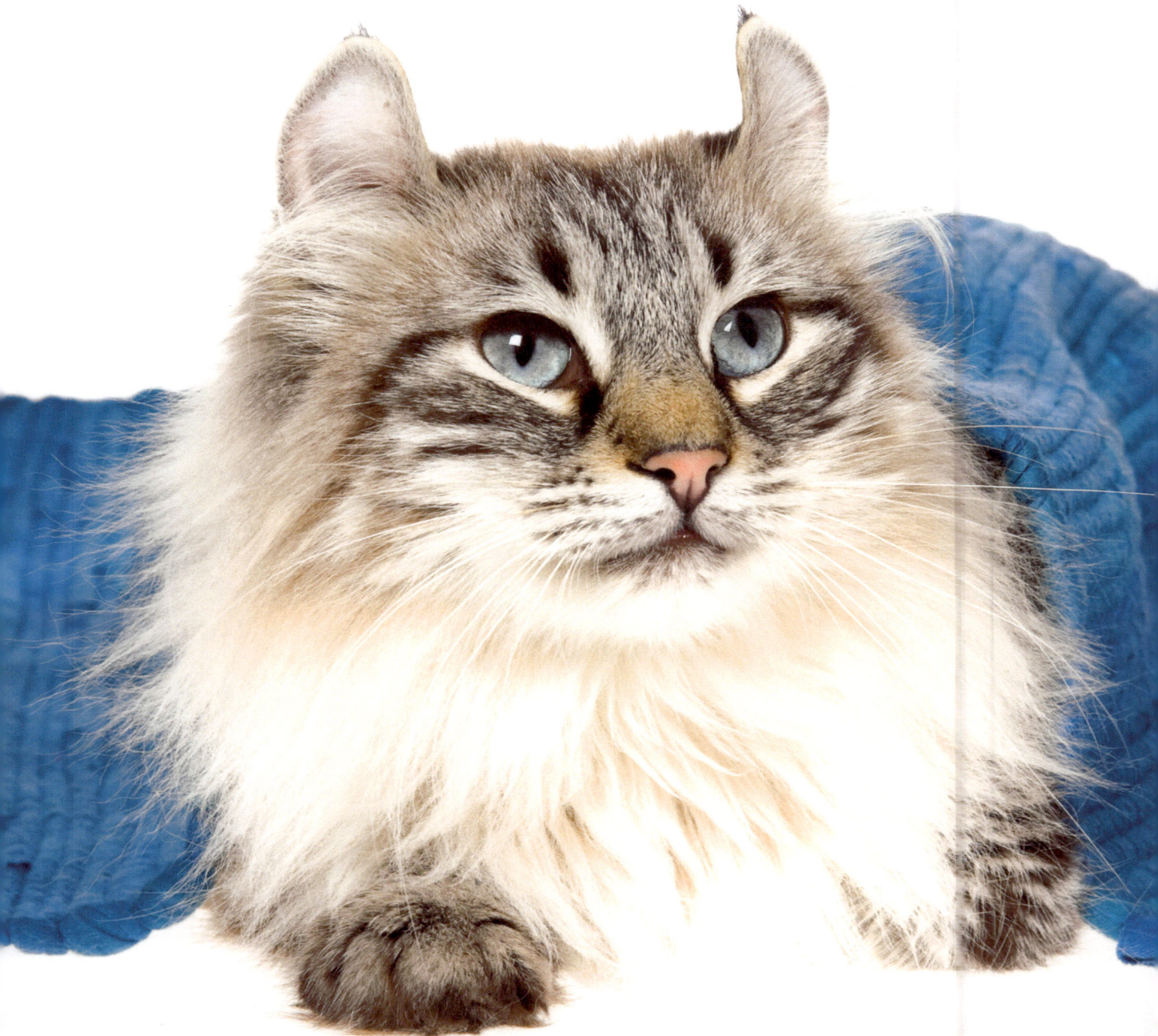

American Shorthair

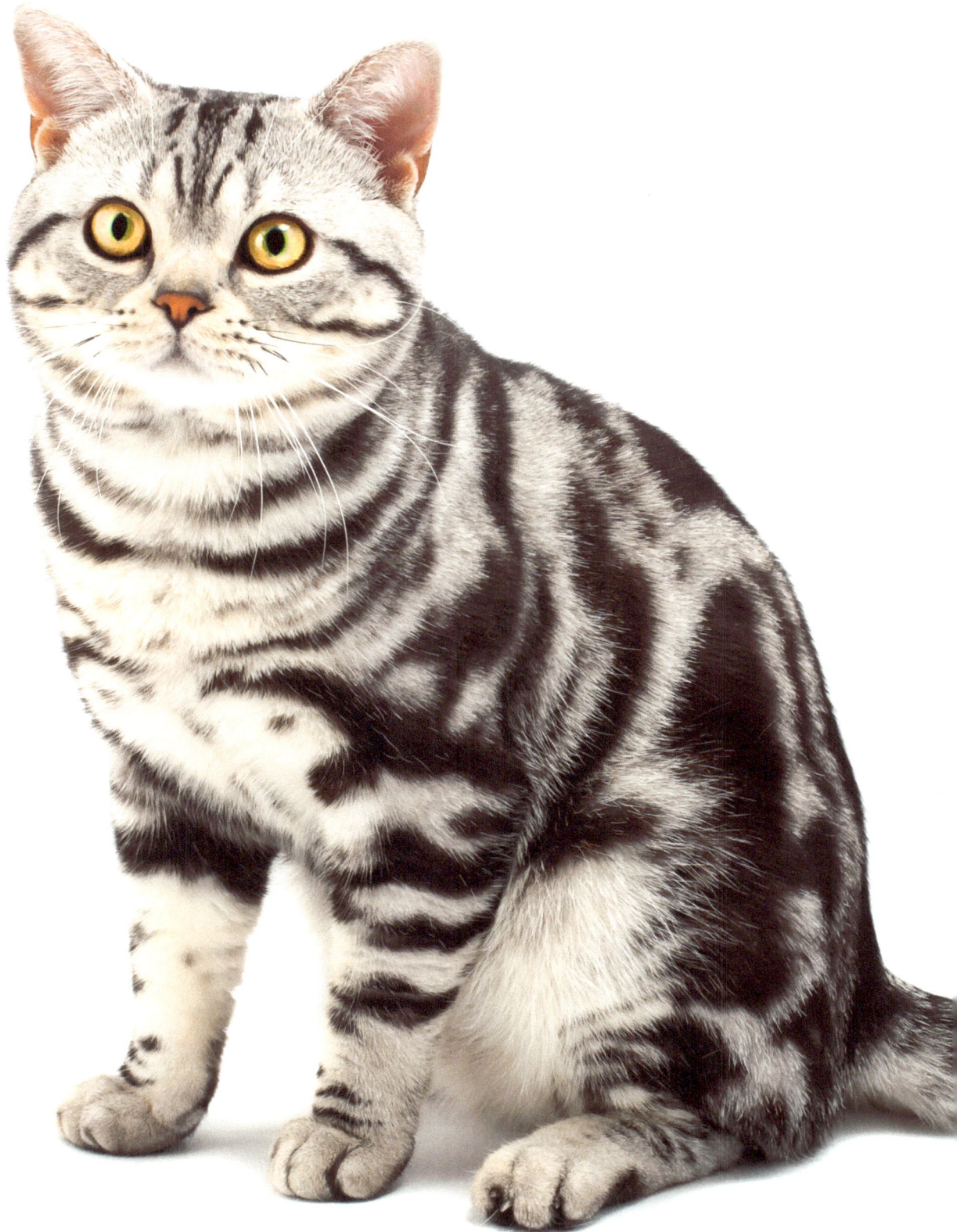

Balinese

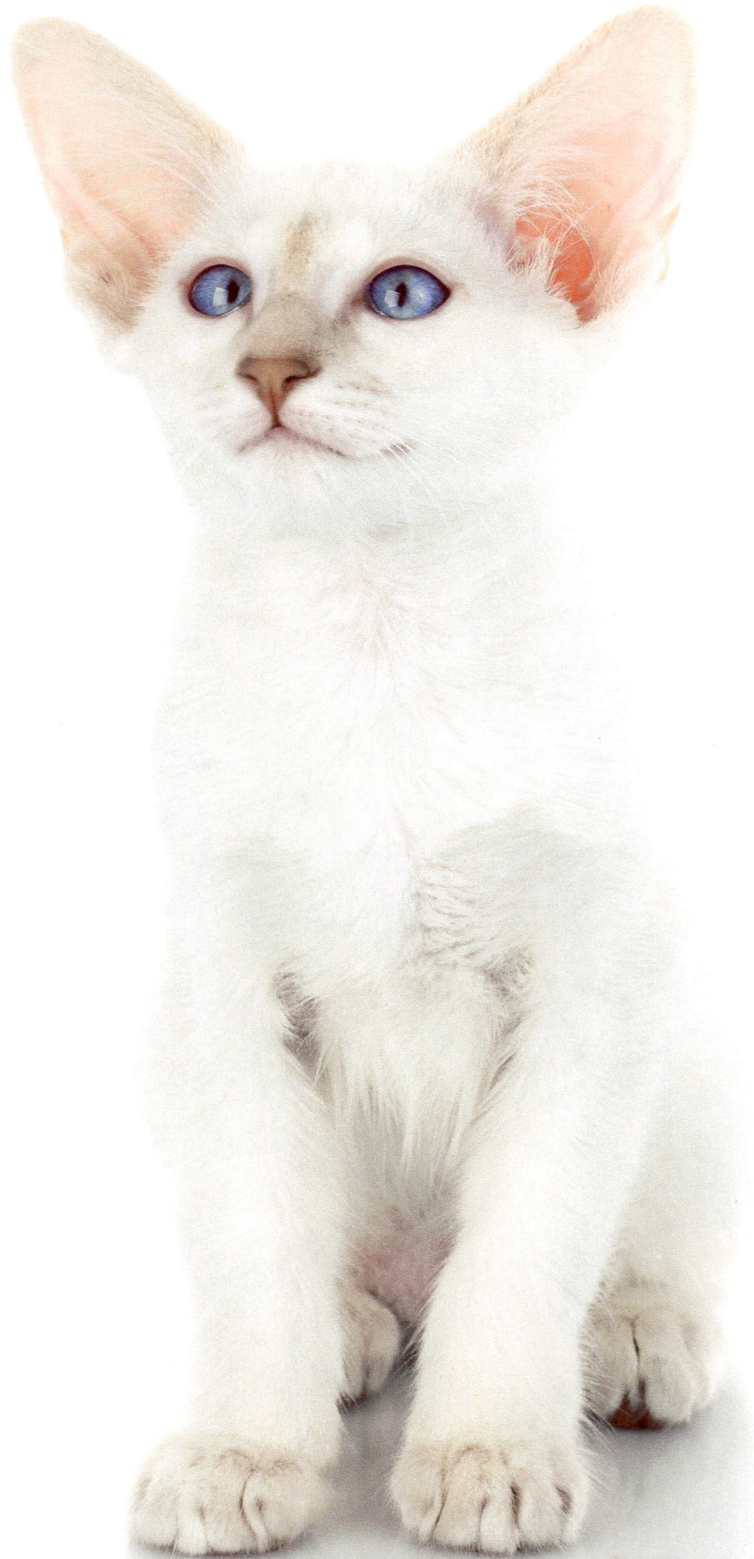

Bengal

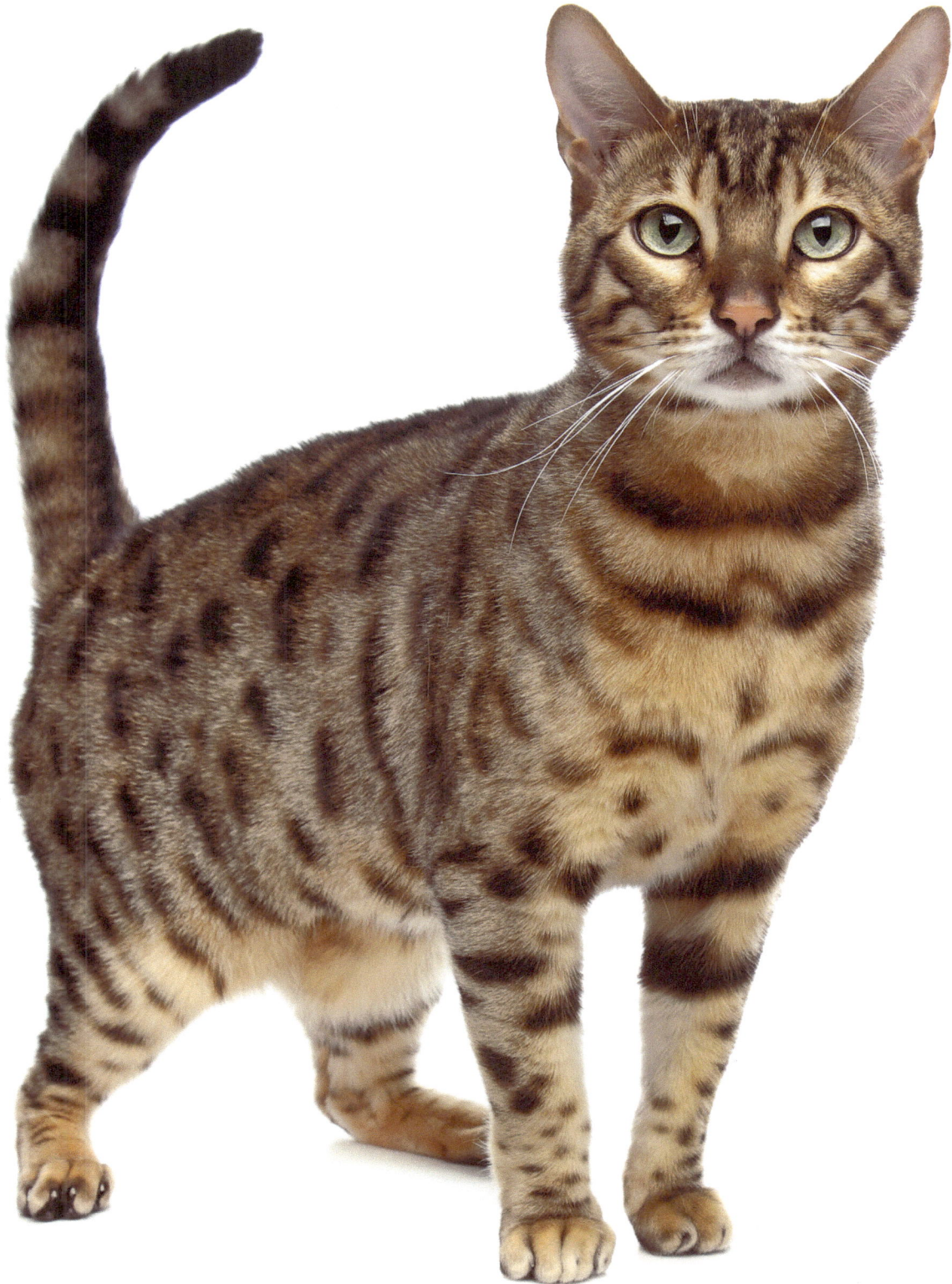

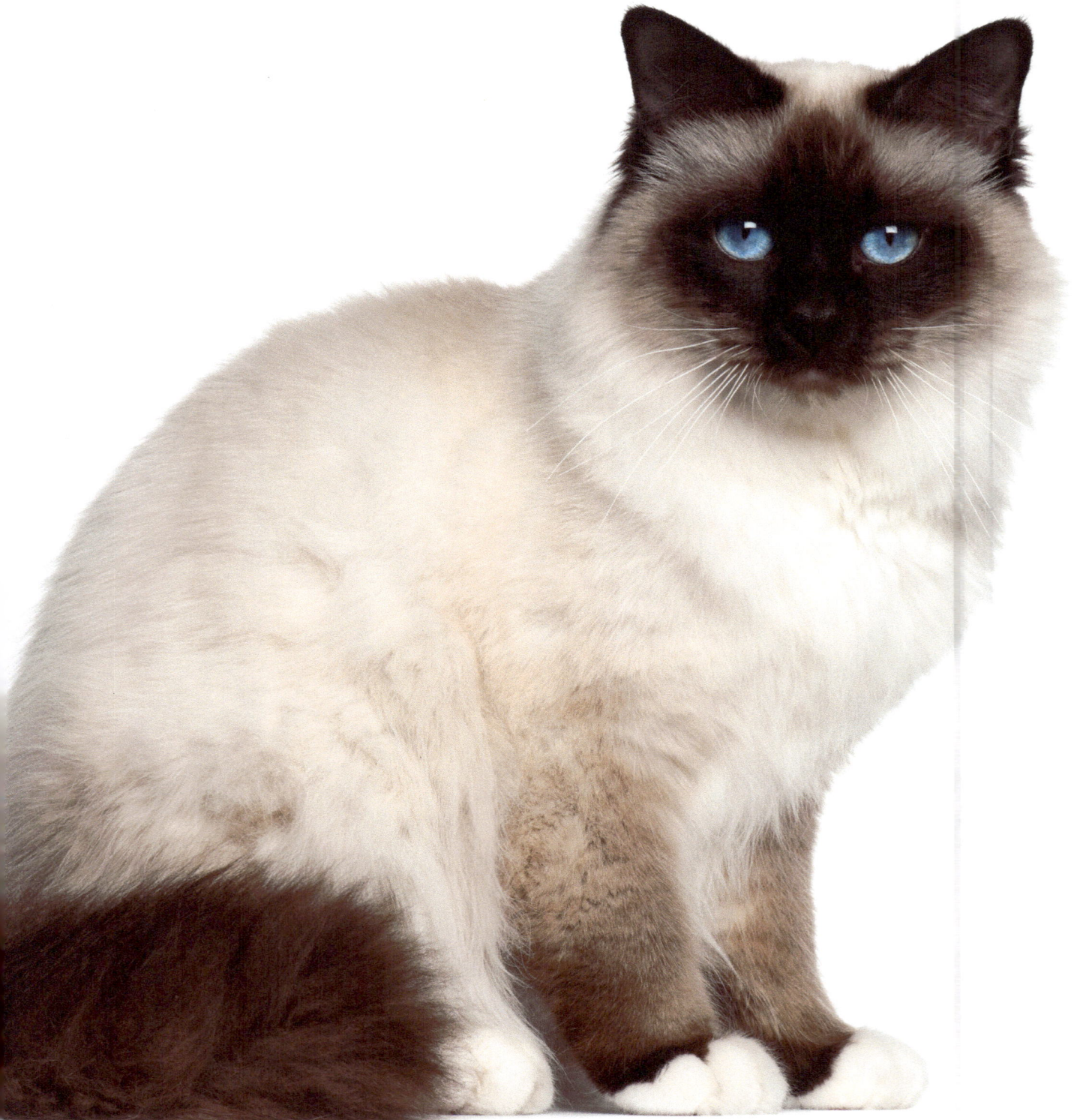

Birman

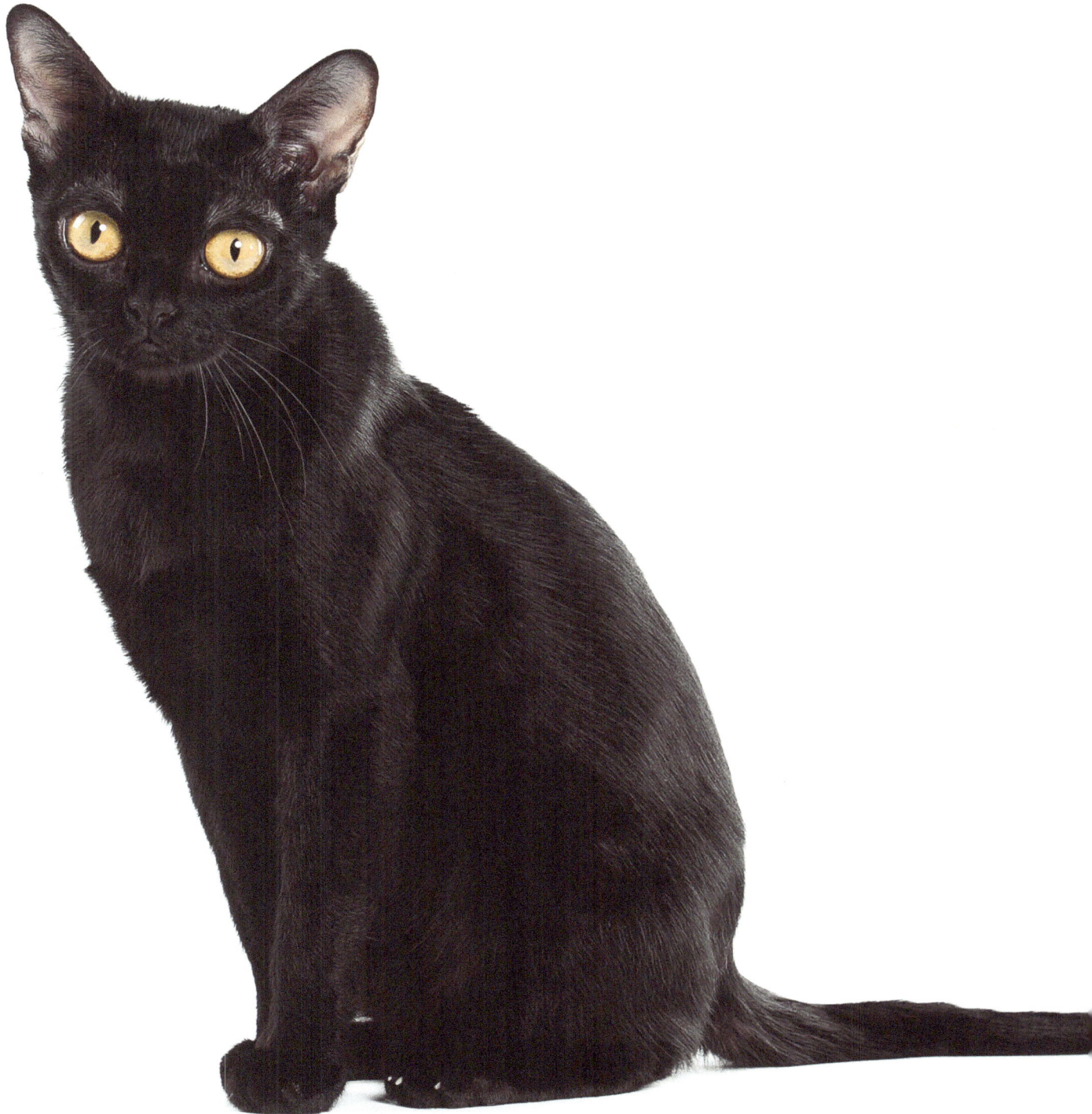

Bombay

British Longhair

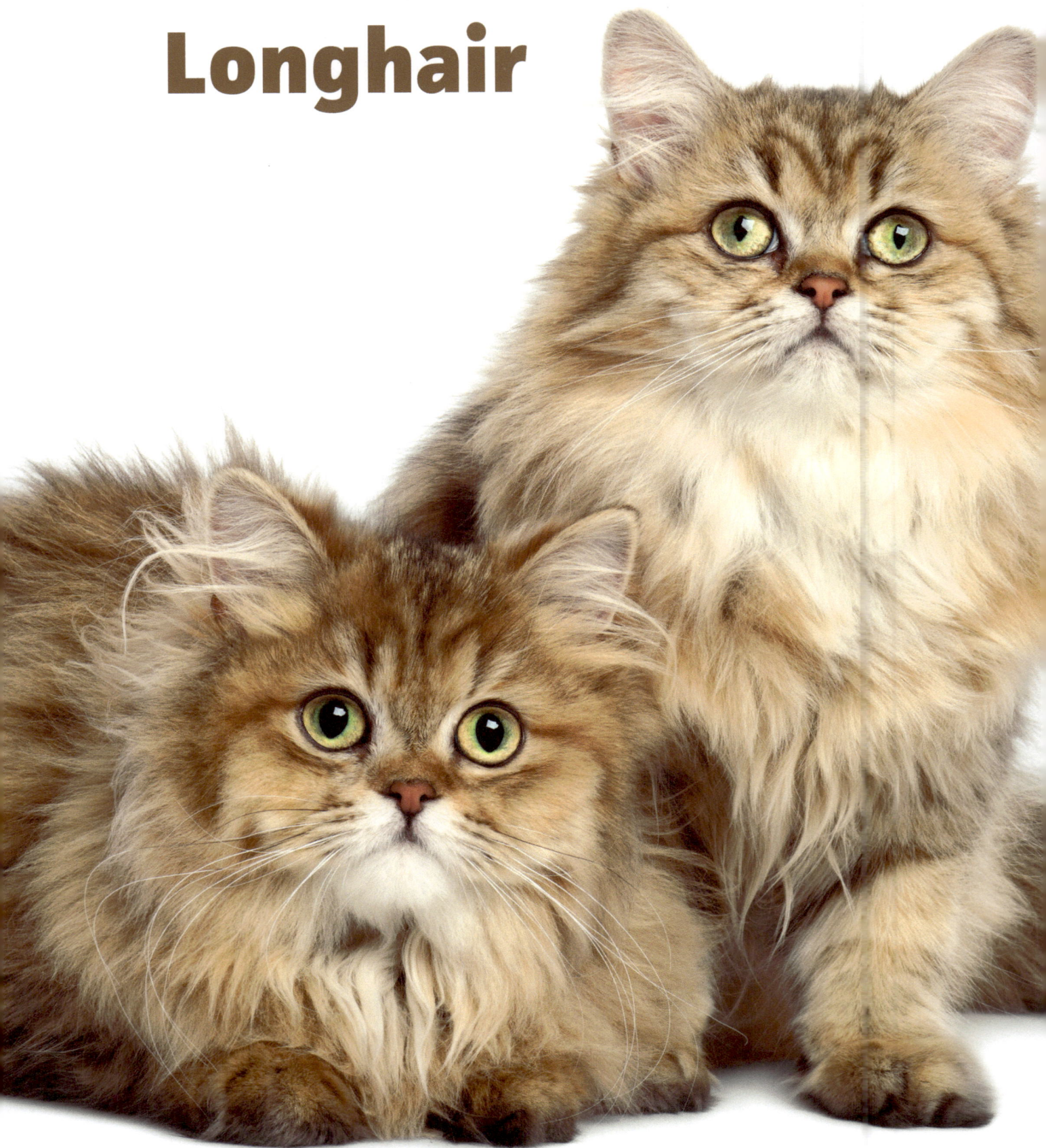

British Shorthair

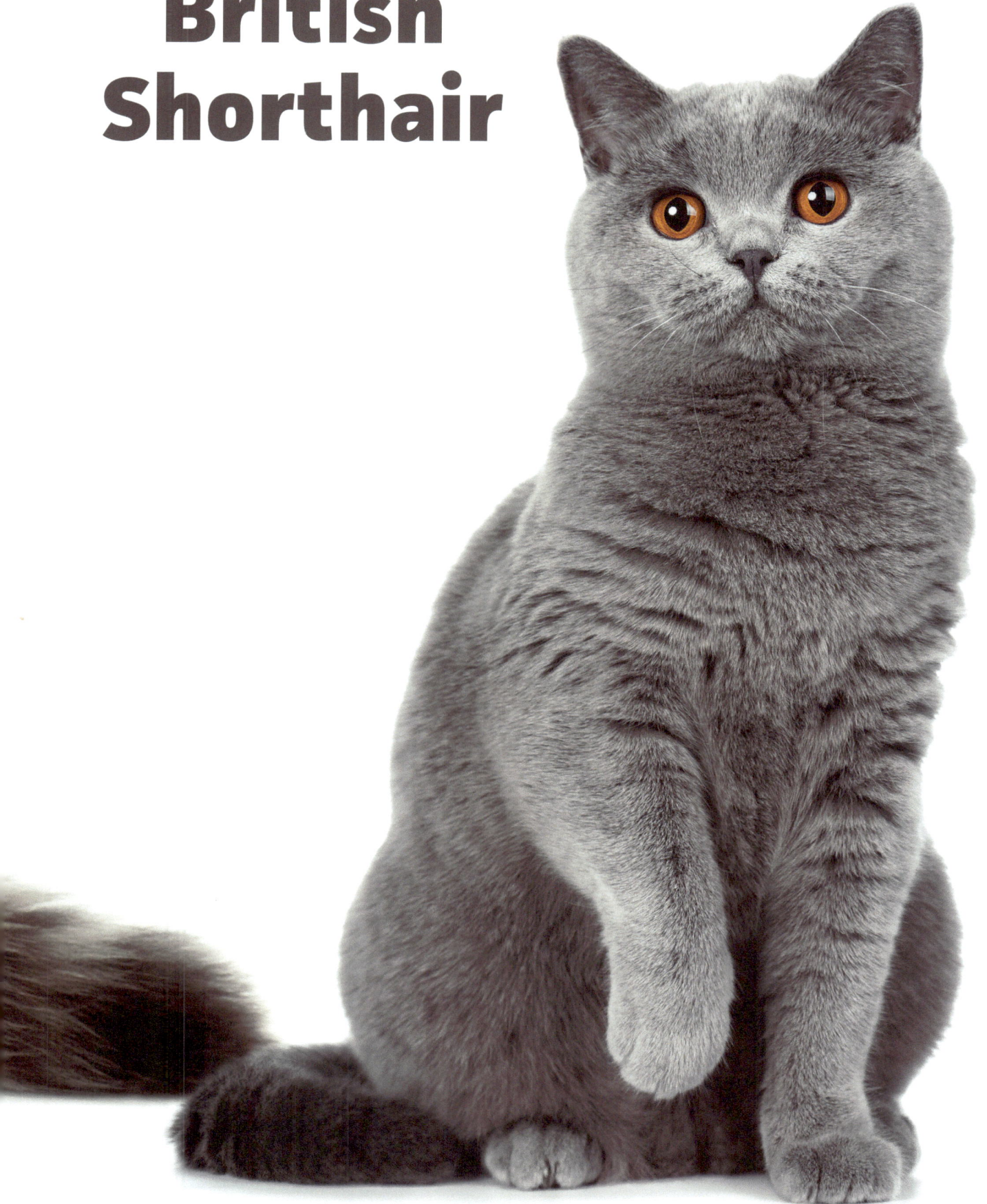

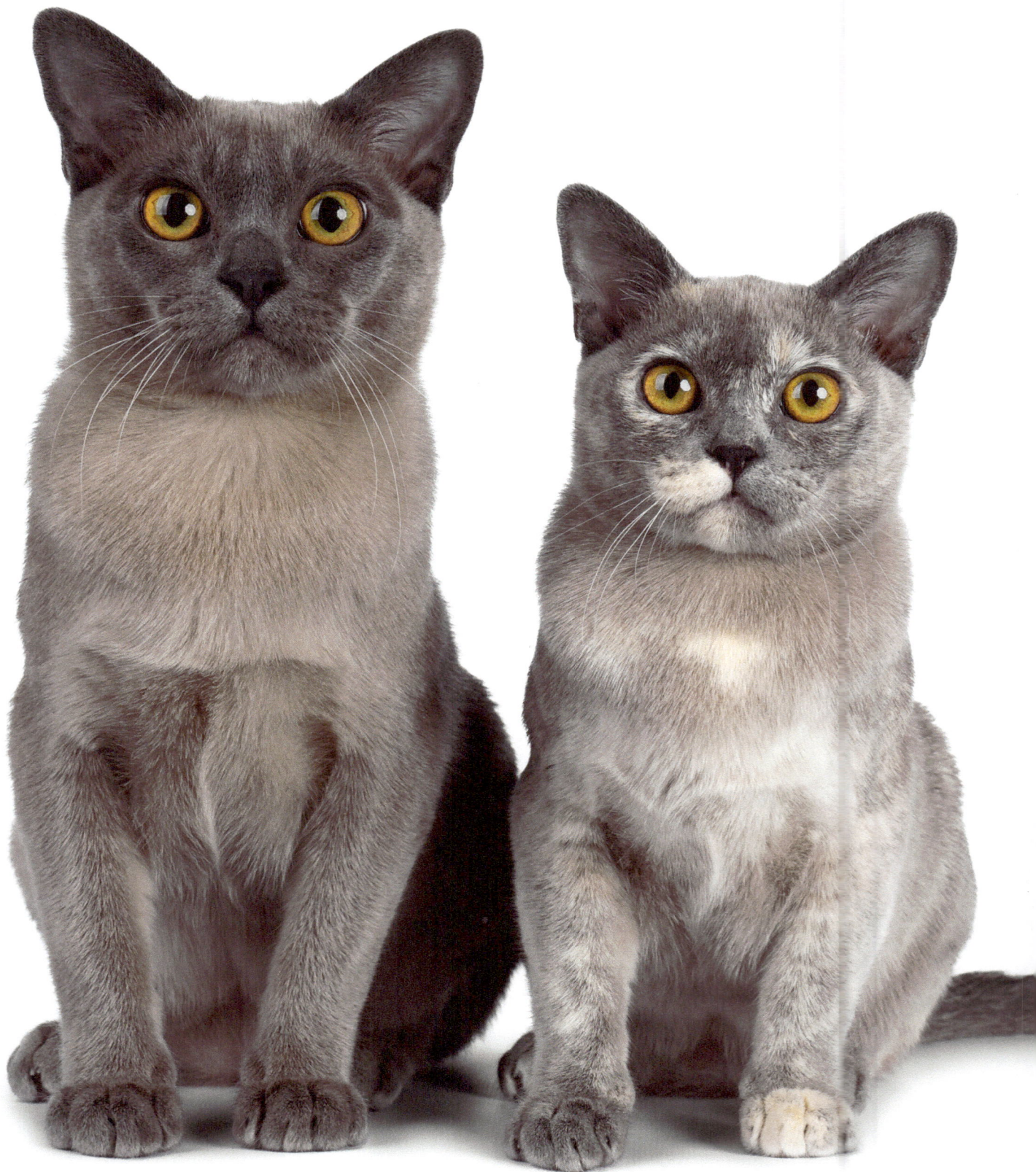

Burmese

Burmilla

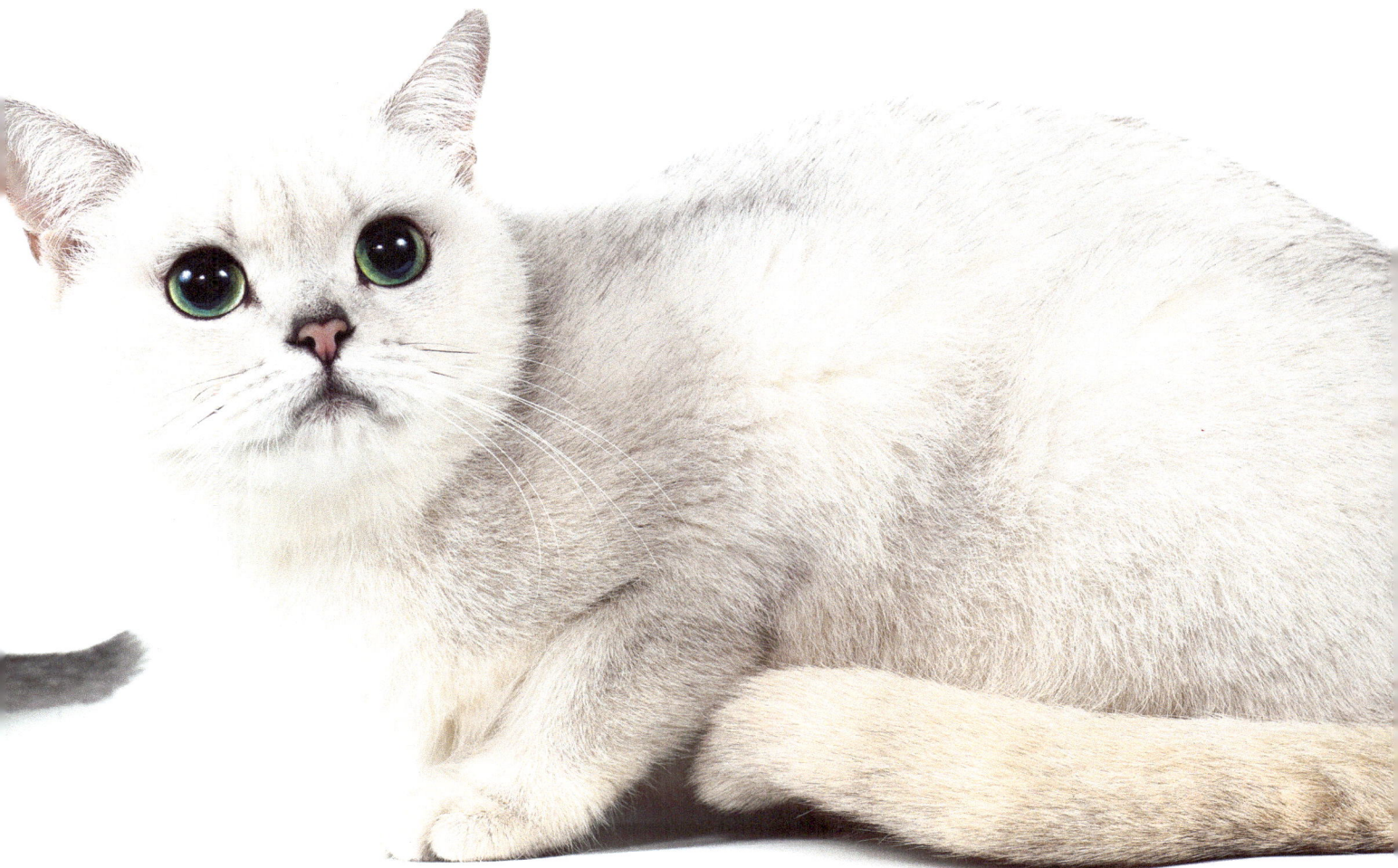

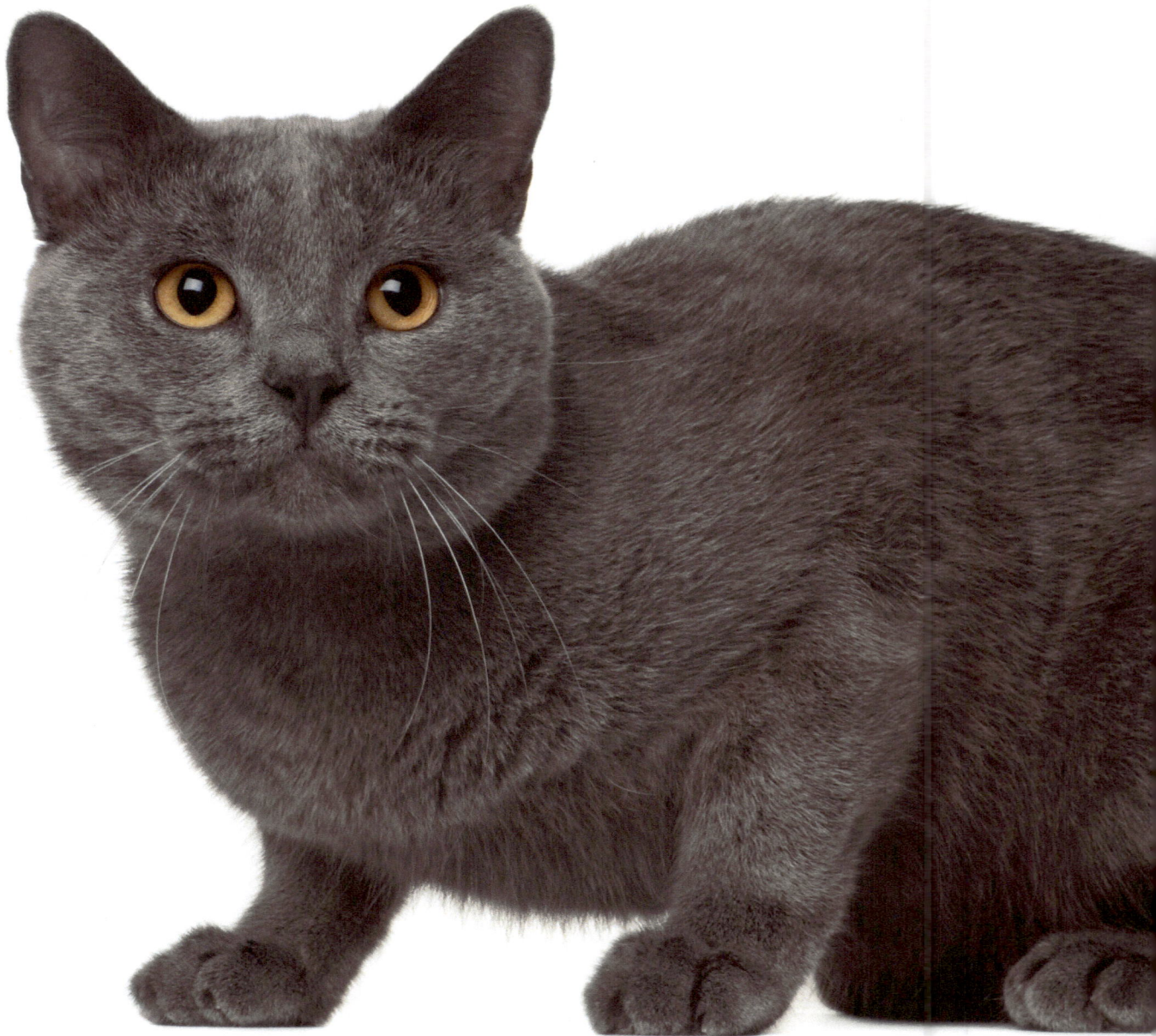

Chartreux

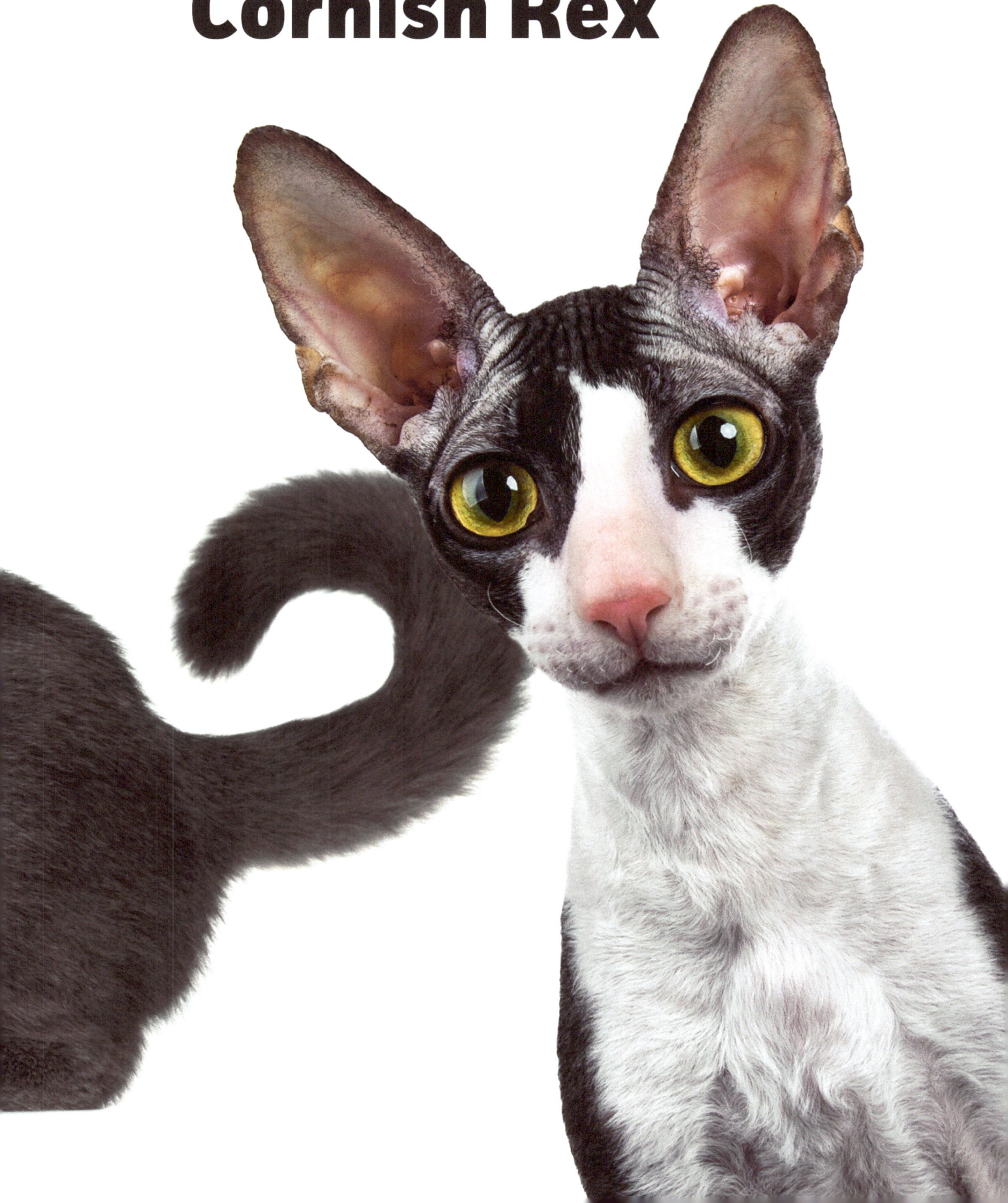

Cornish Rex

Devon Rex

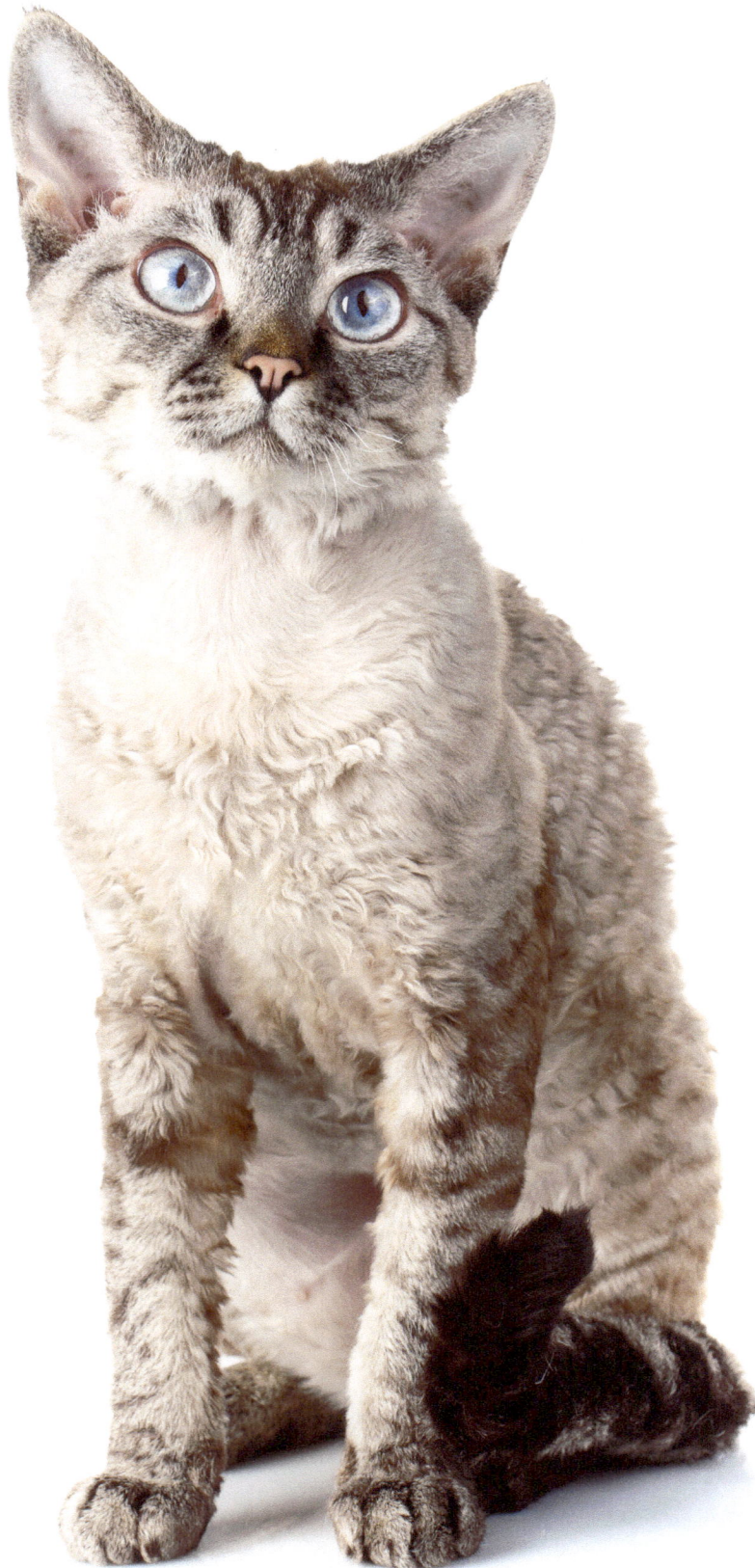
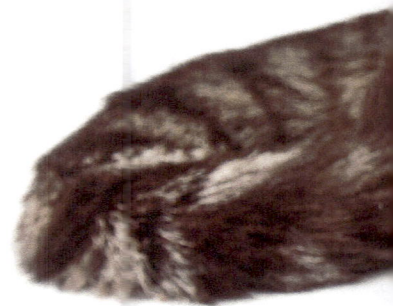

Domestic Shorthair

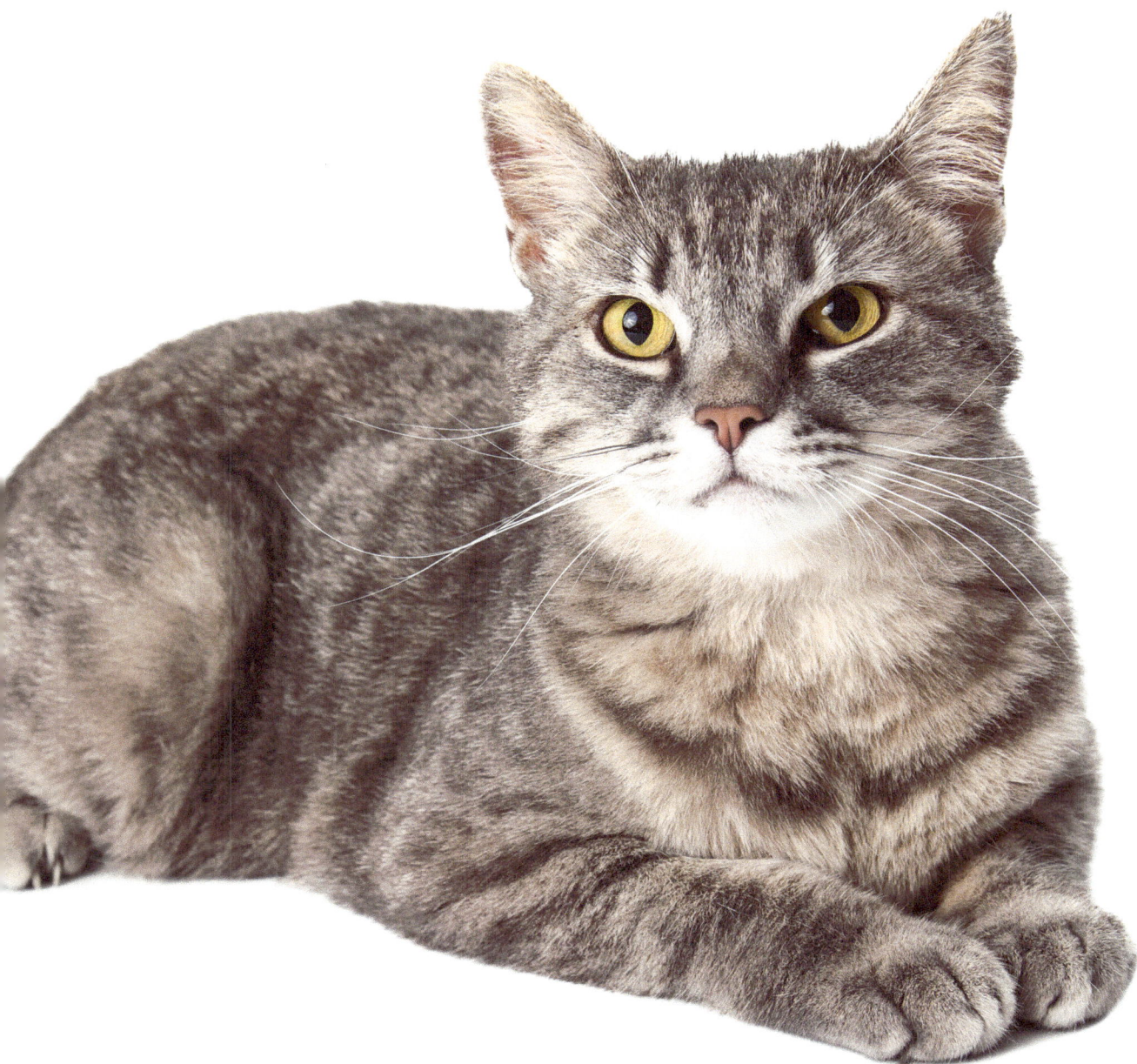

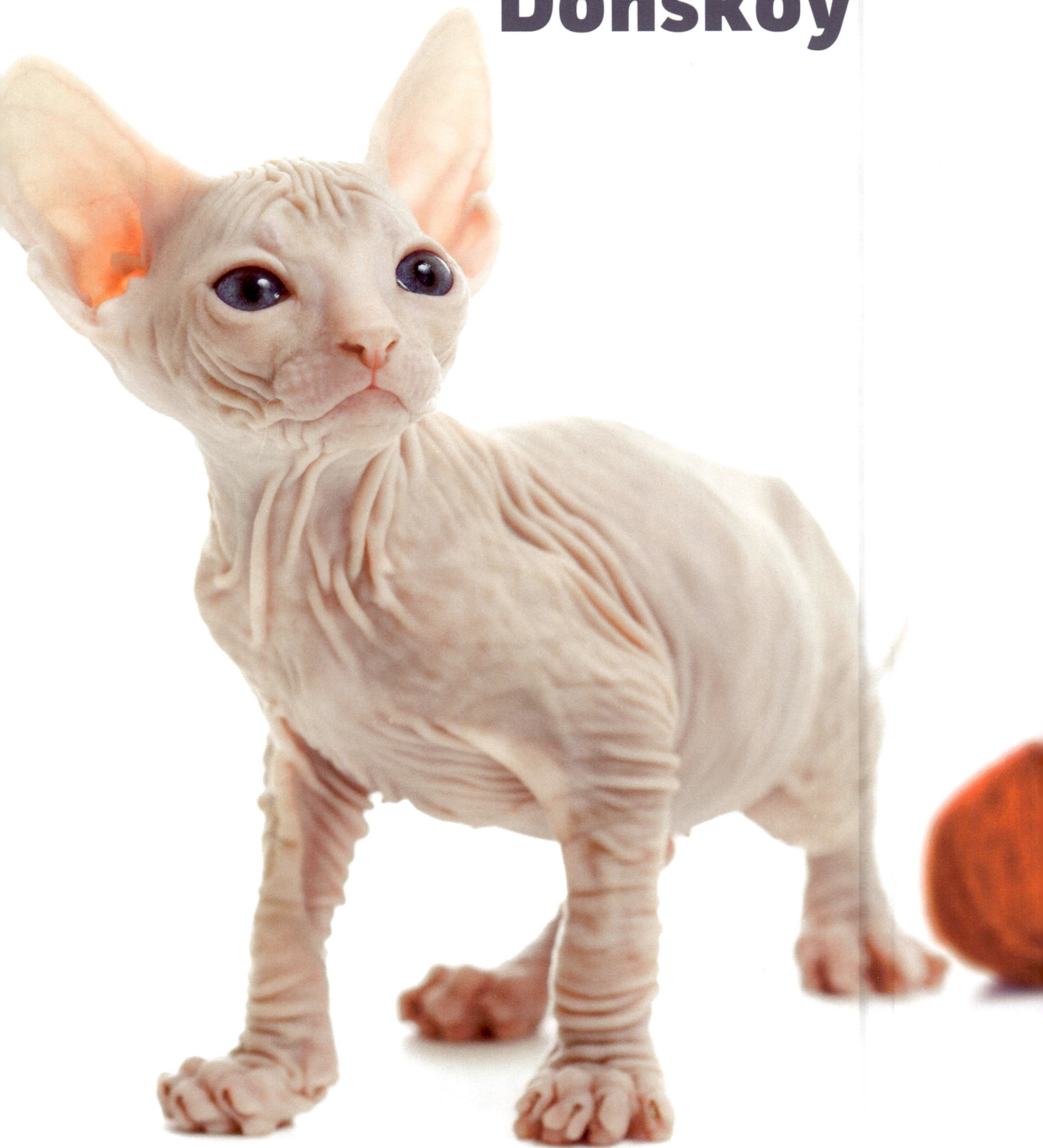

Donskoy

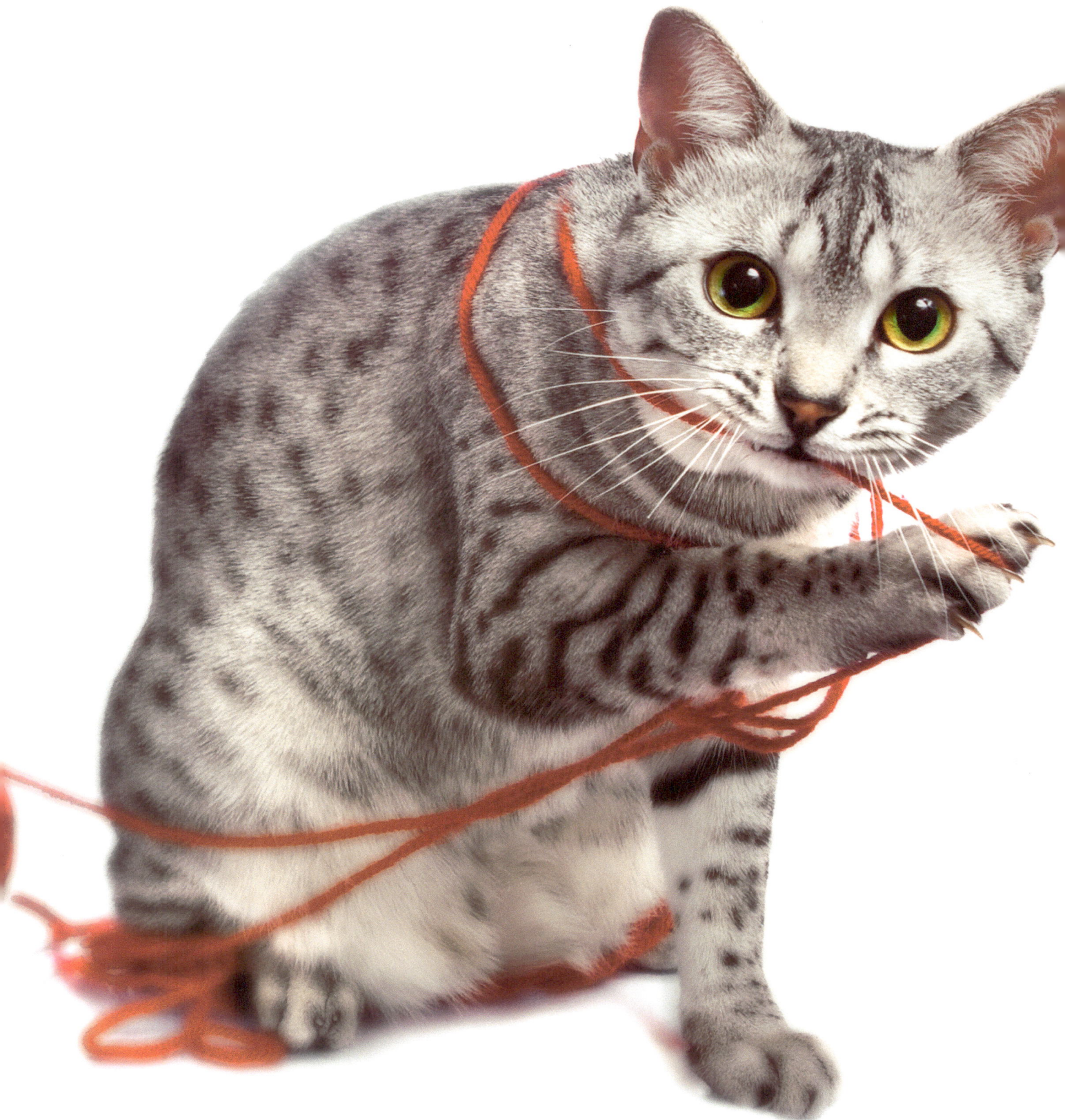

Egyptian Mau

Exotic Shorthair

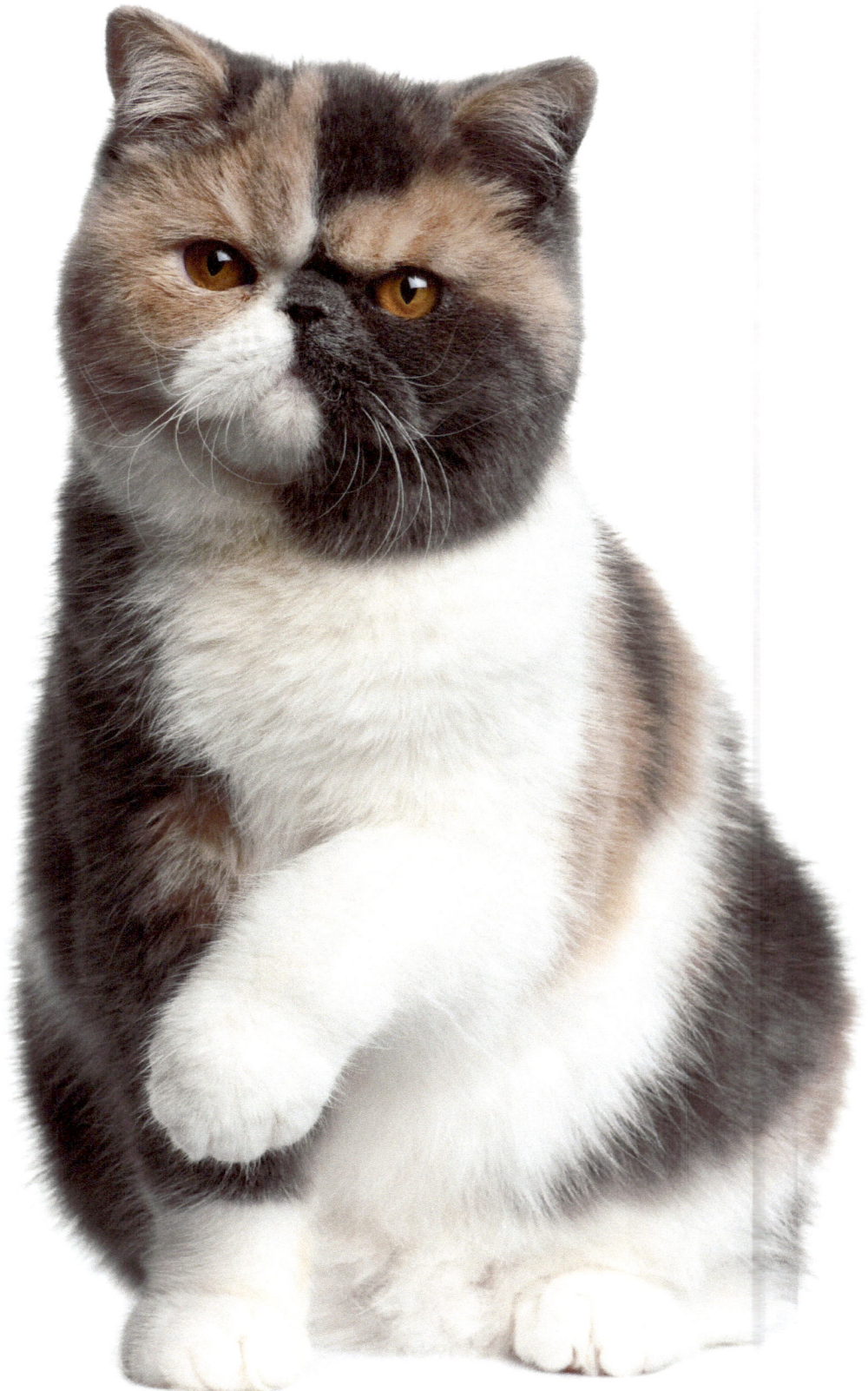

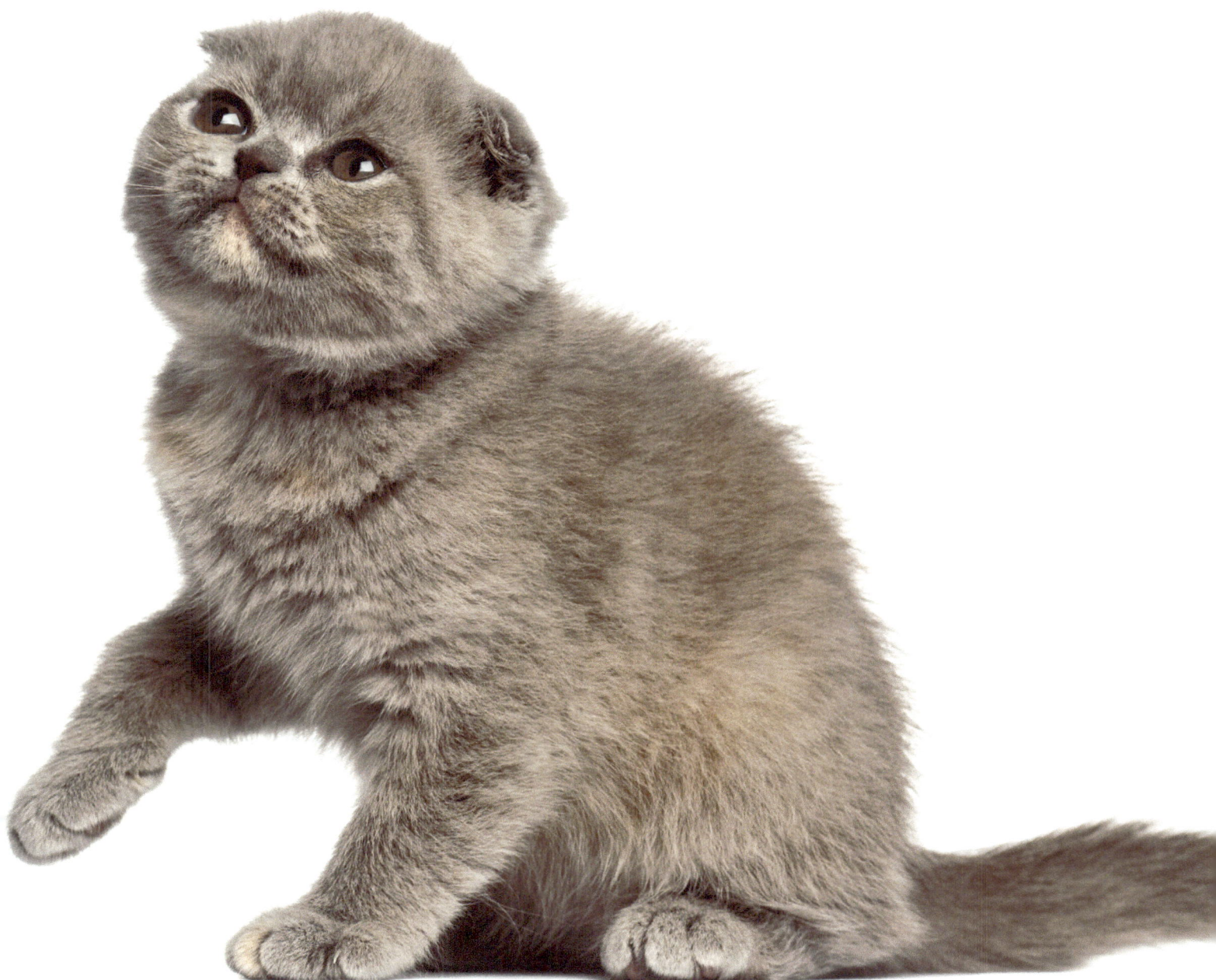

Foldex

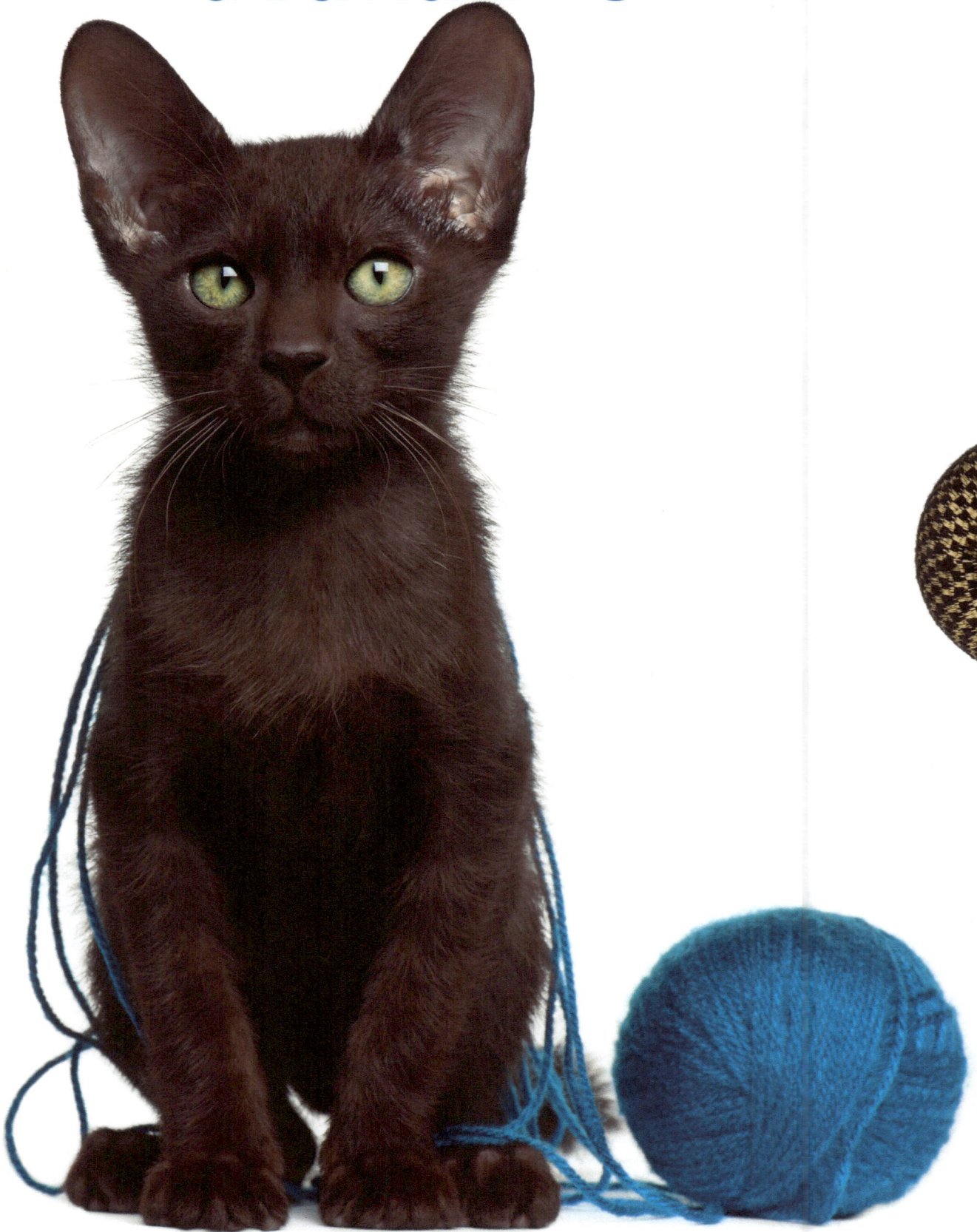

Havana Brown

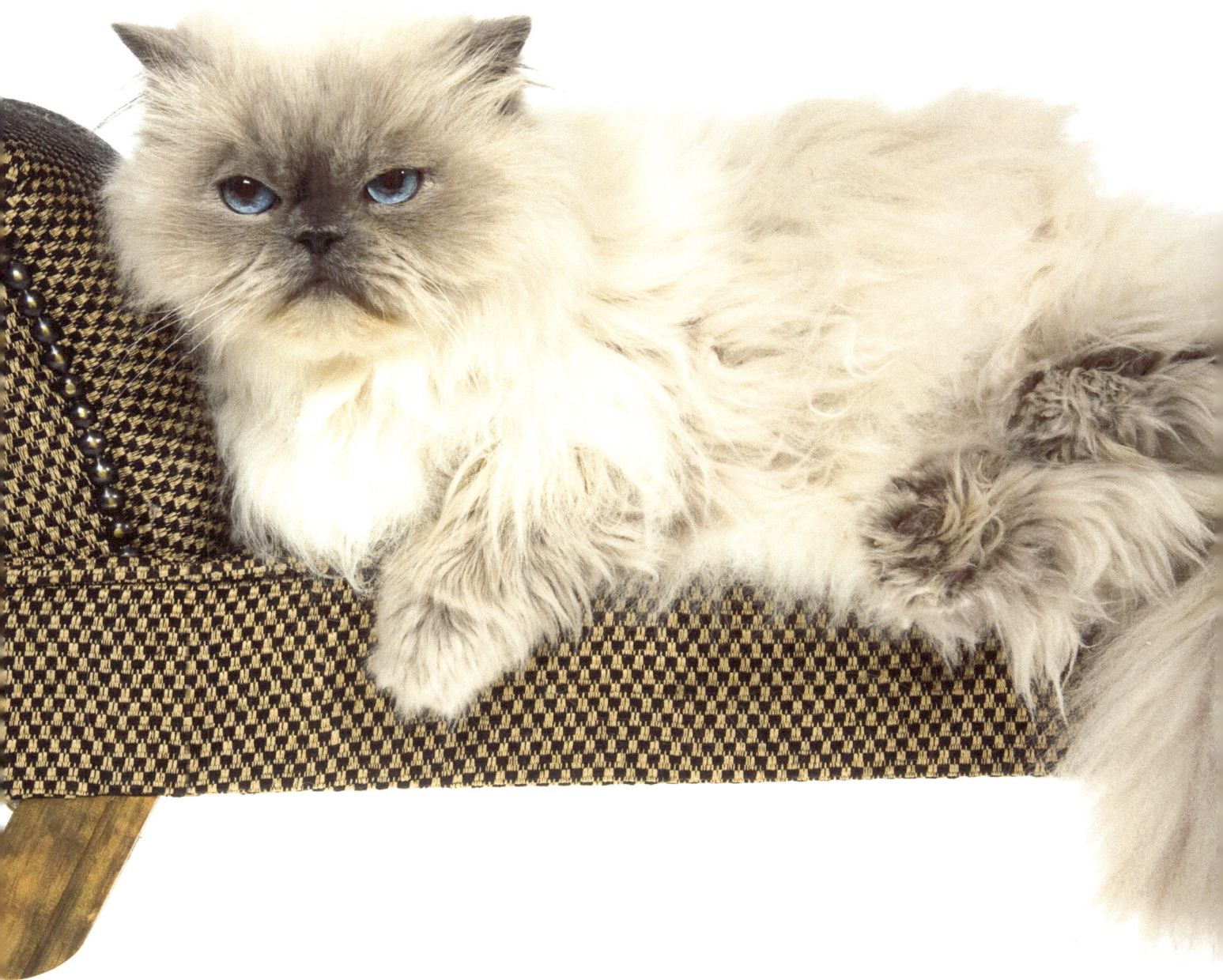

Himalayan

Japanese Bobtail

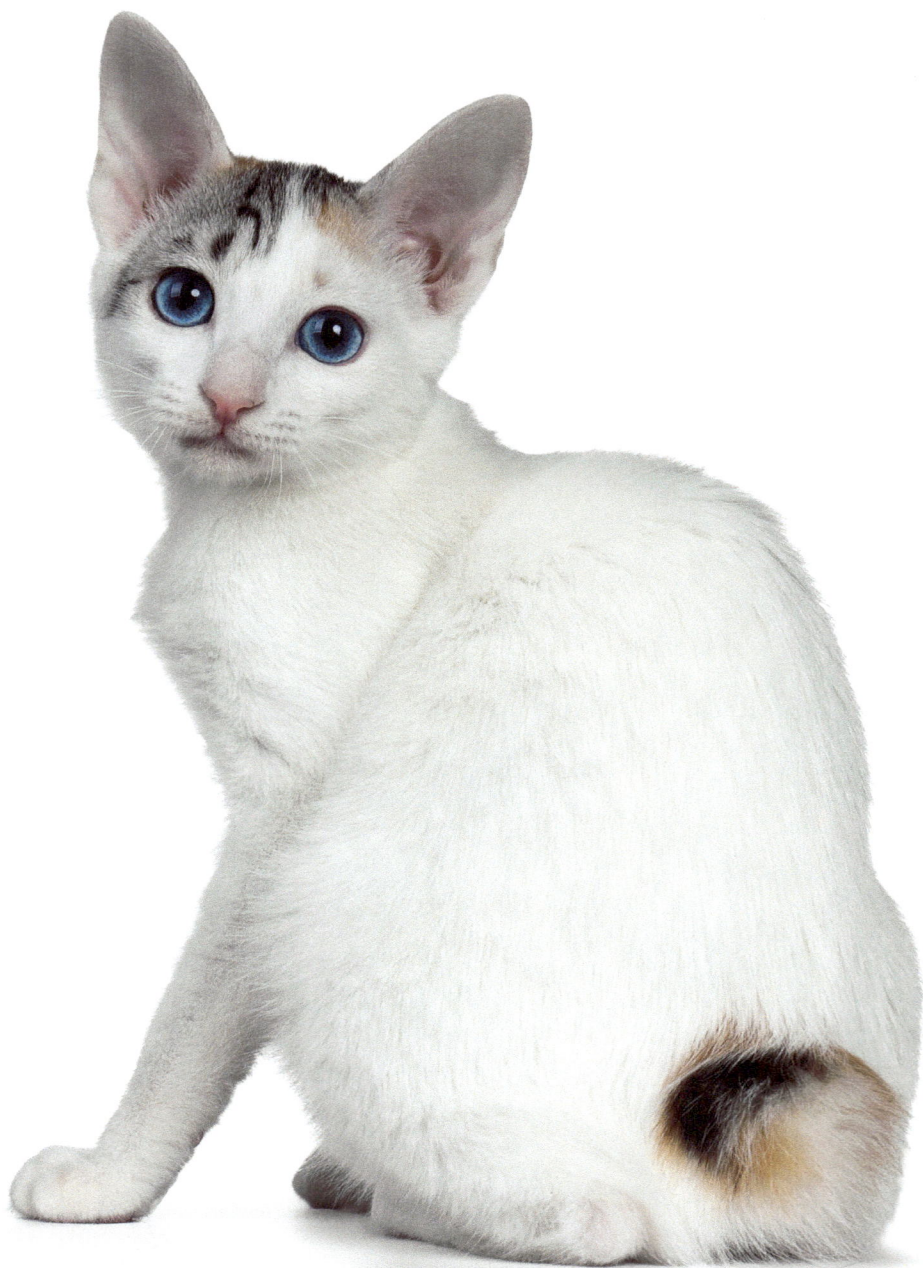

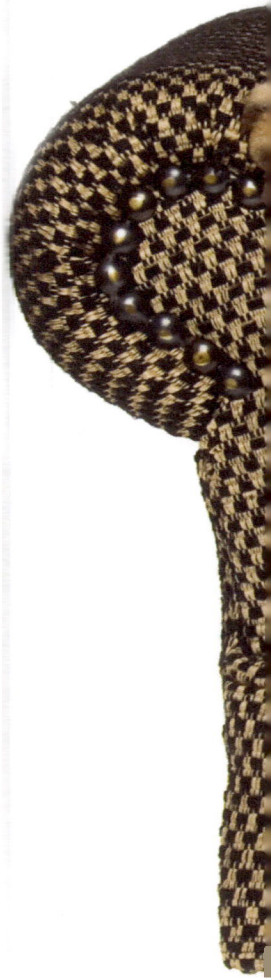

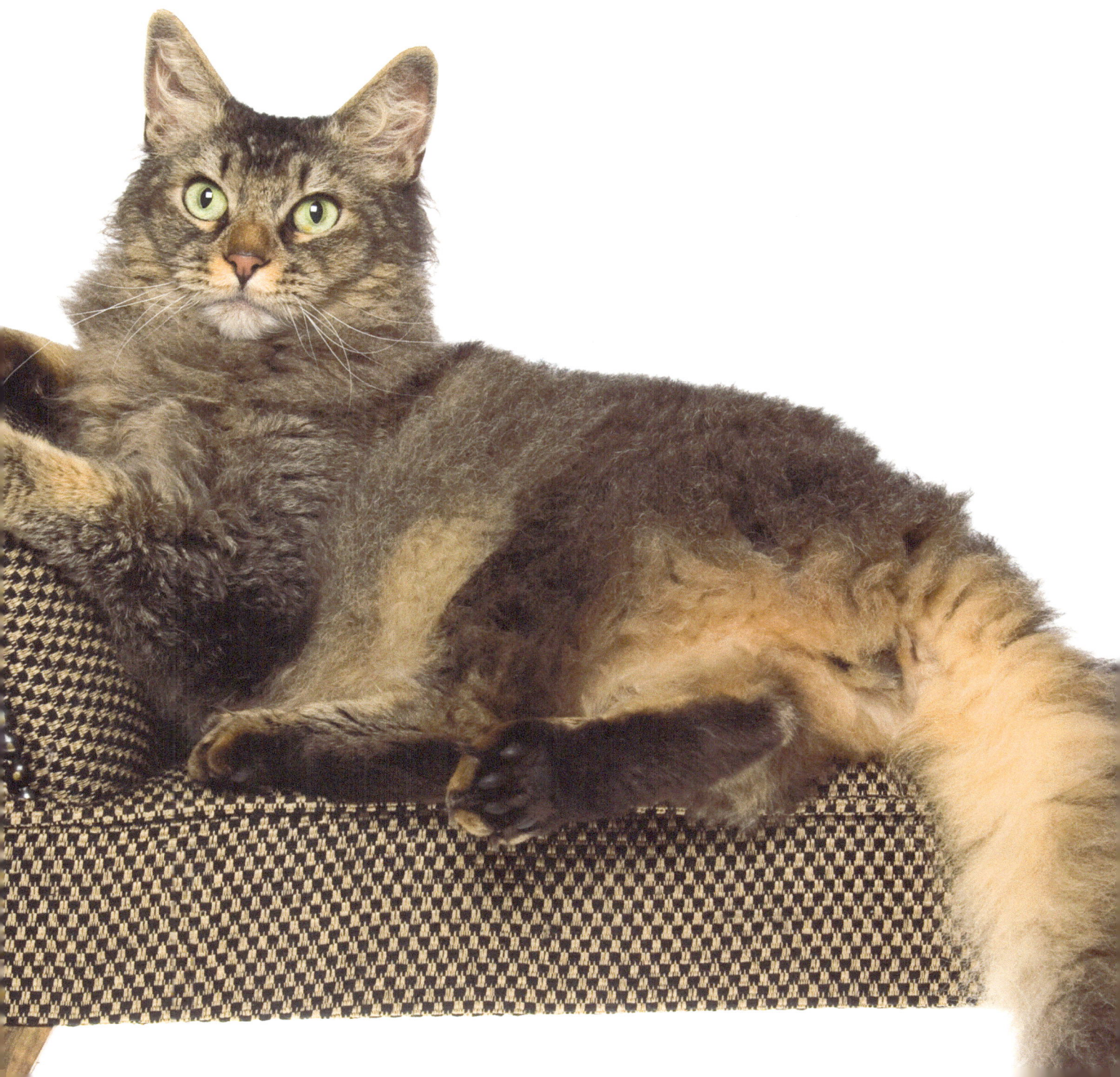

LaPerm

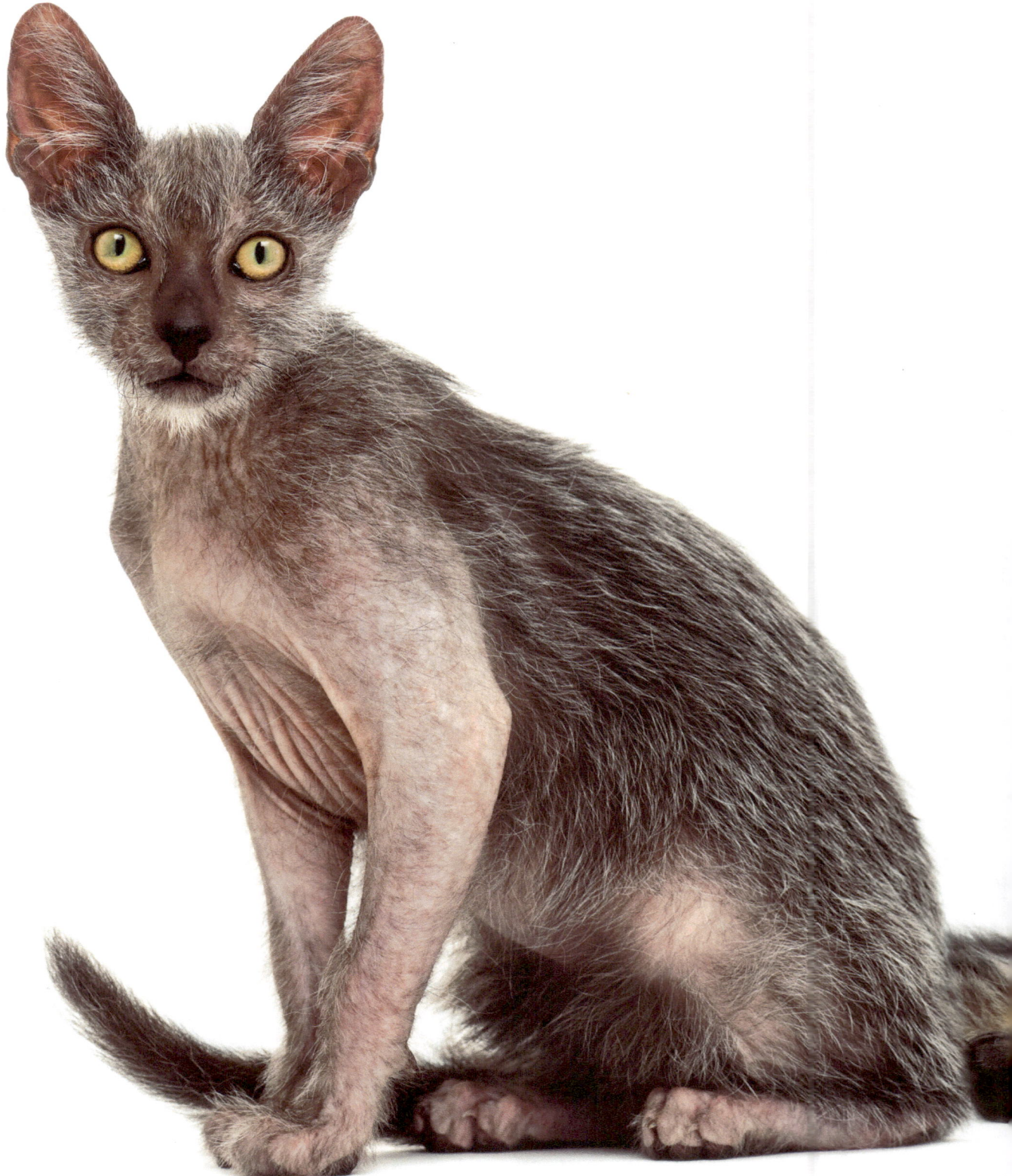

Lykoi

Maine Coon

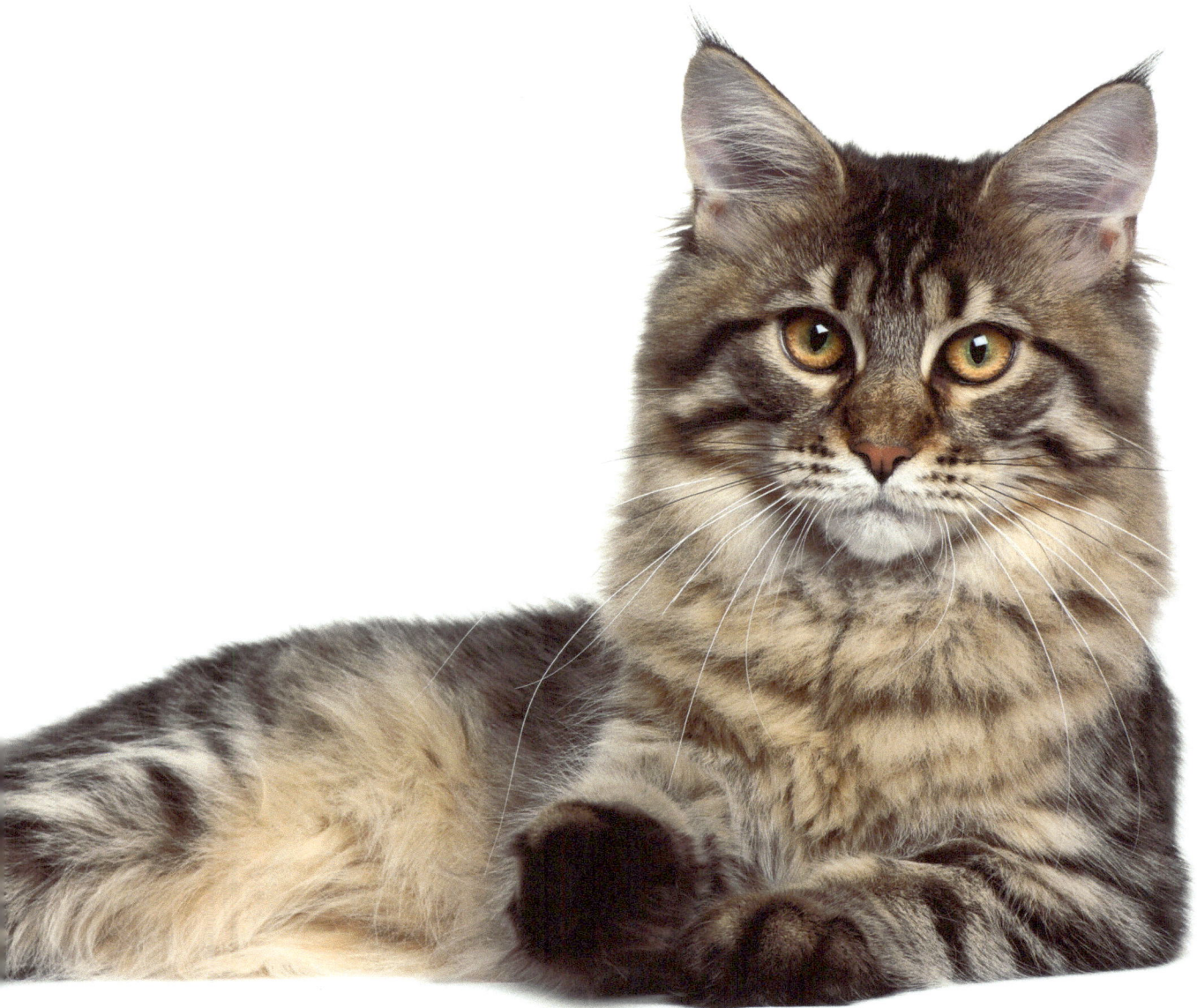

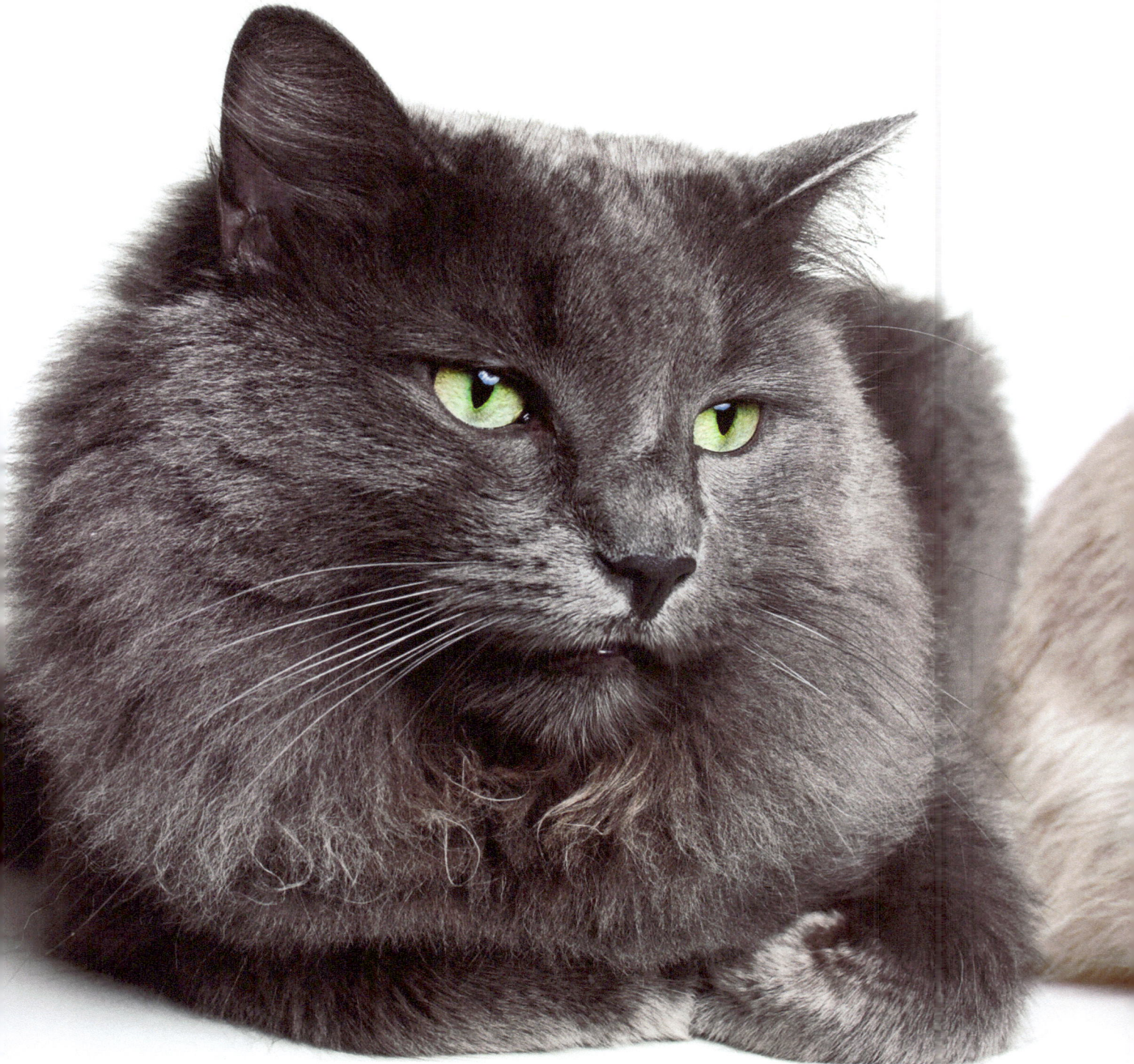

Munchkin

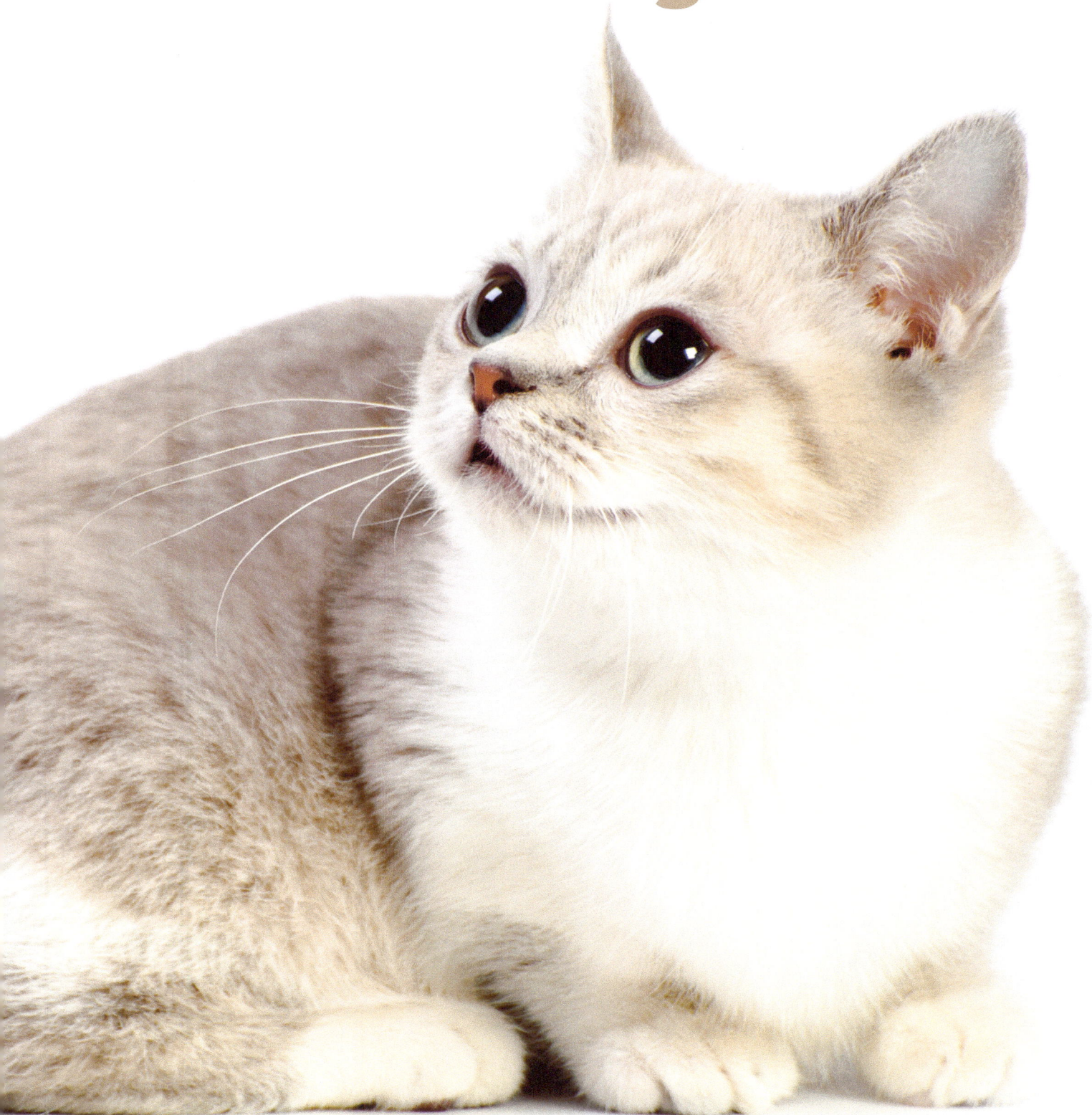

Nebelung

Norwegian Forest

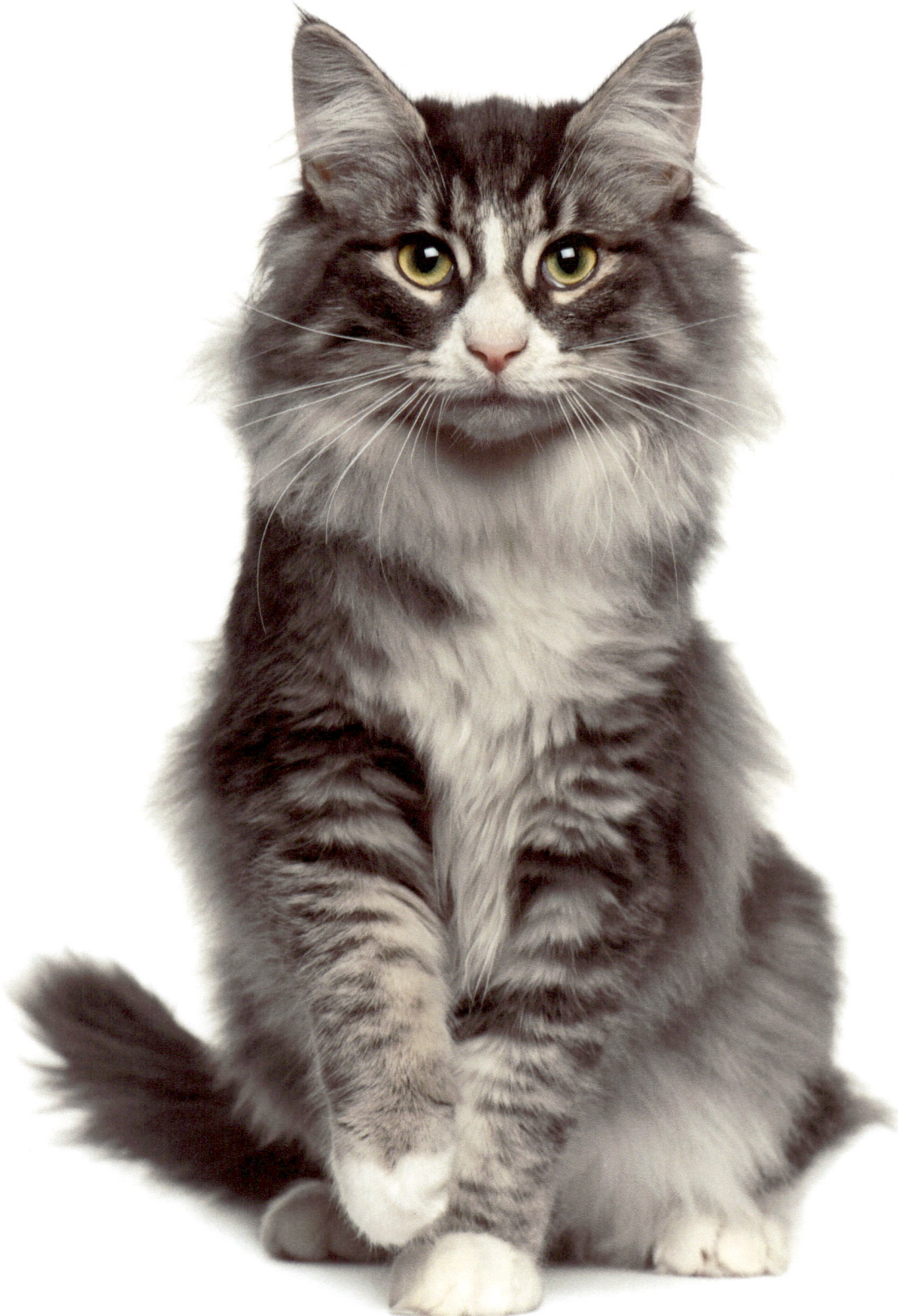

Ocicat

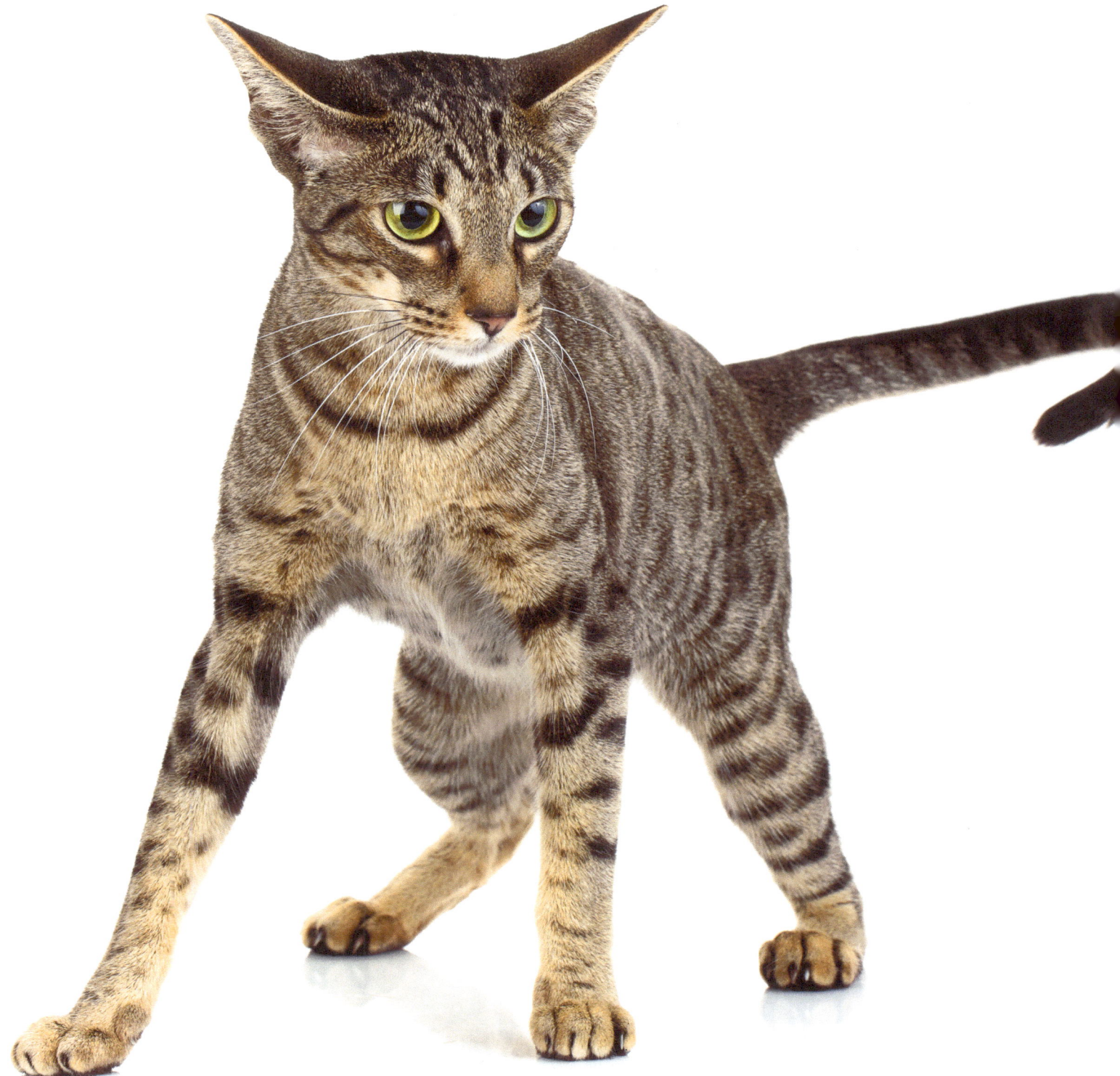

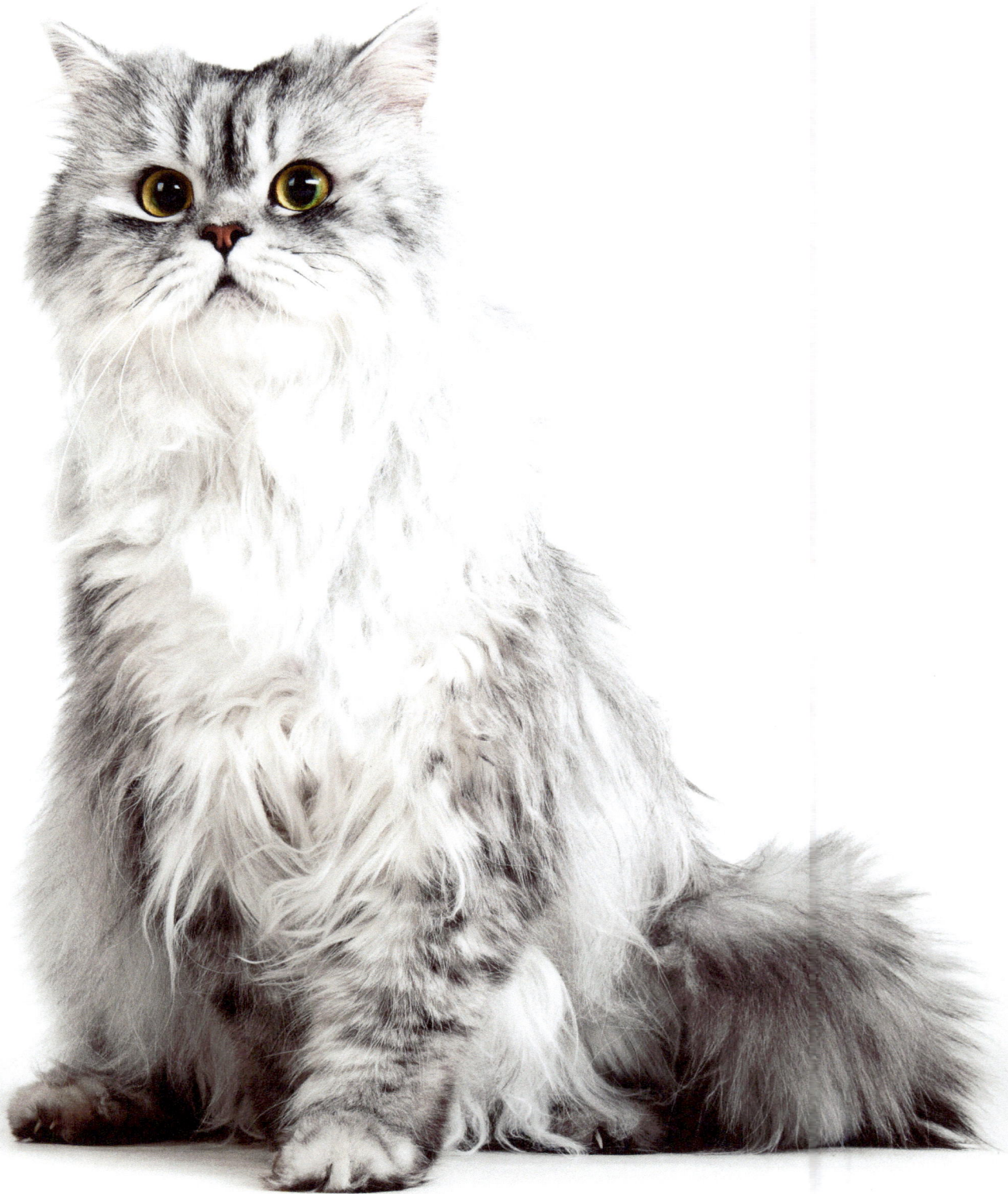

Persian

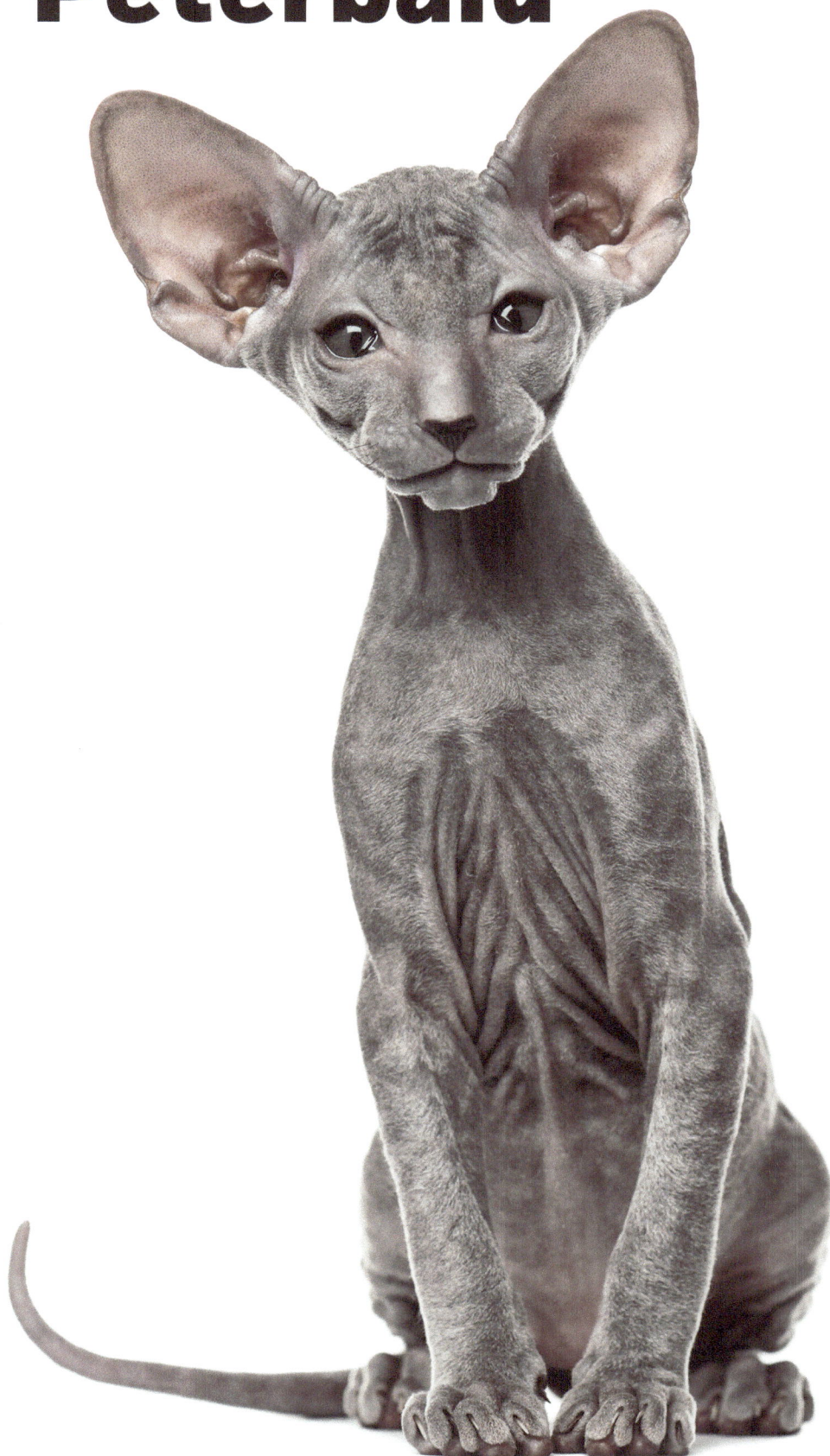

Peterbald

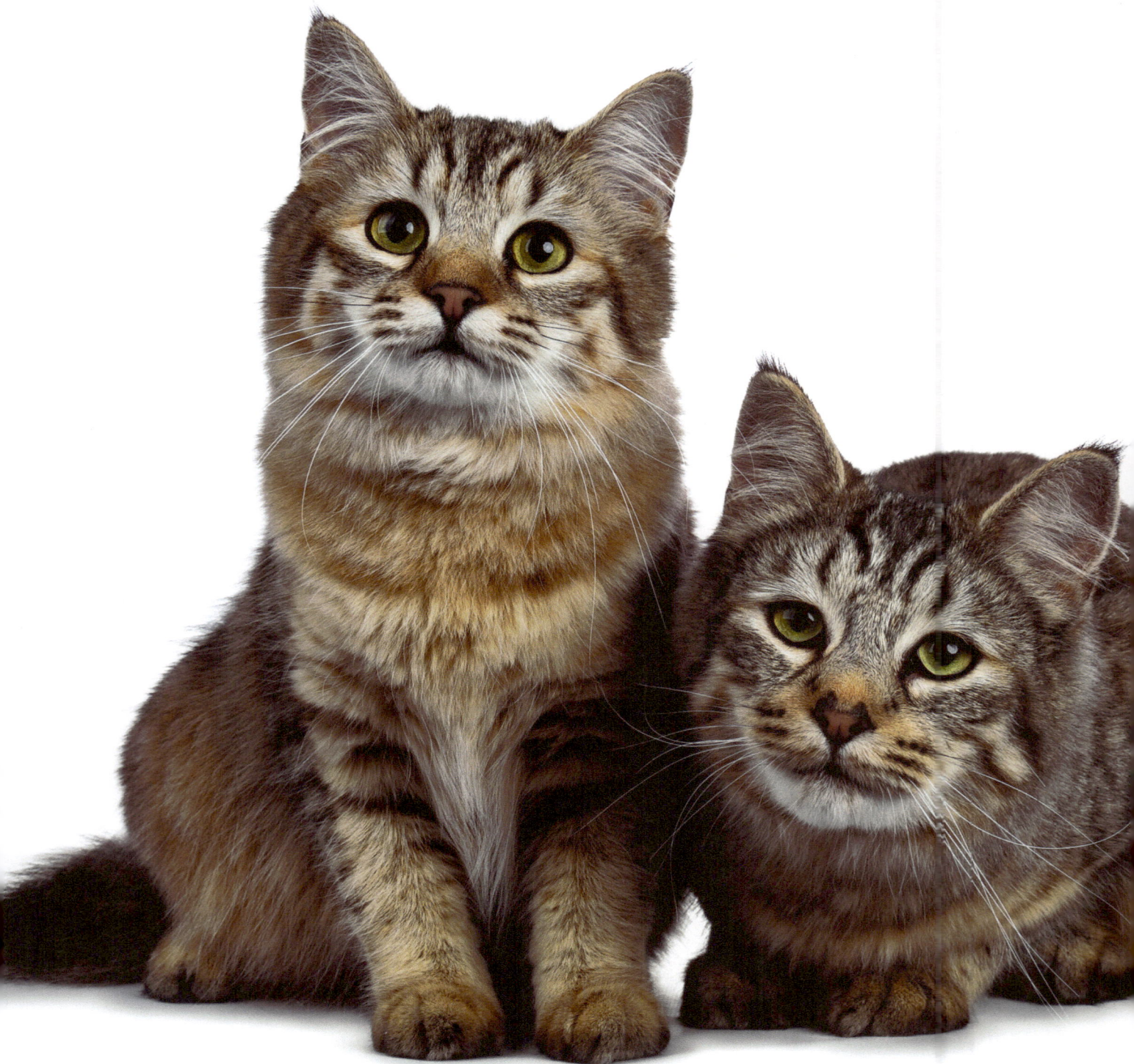

Pixie Bob

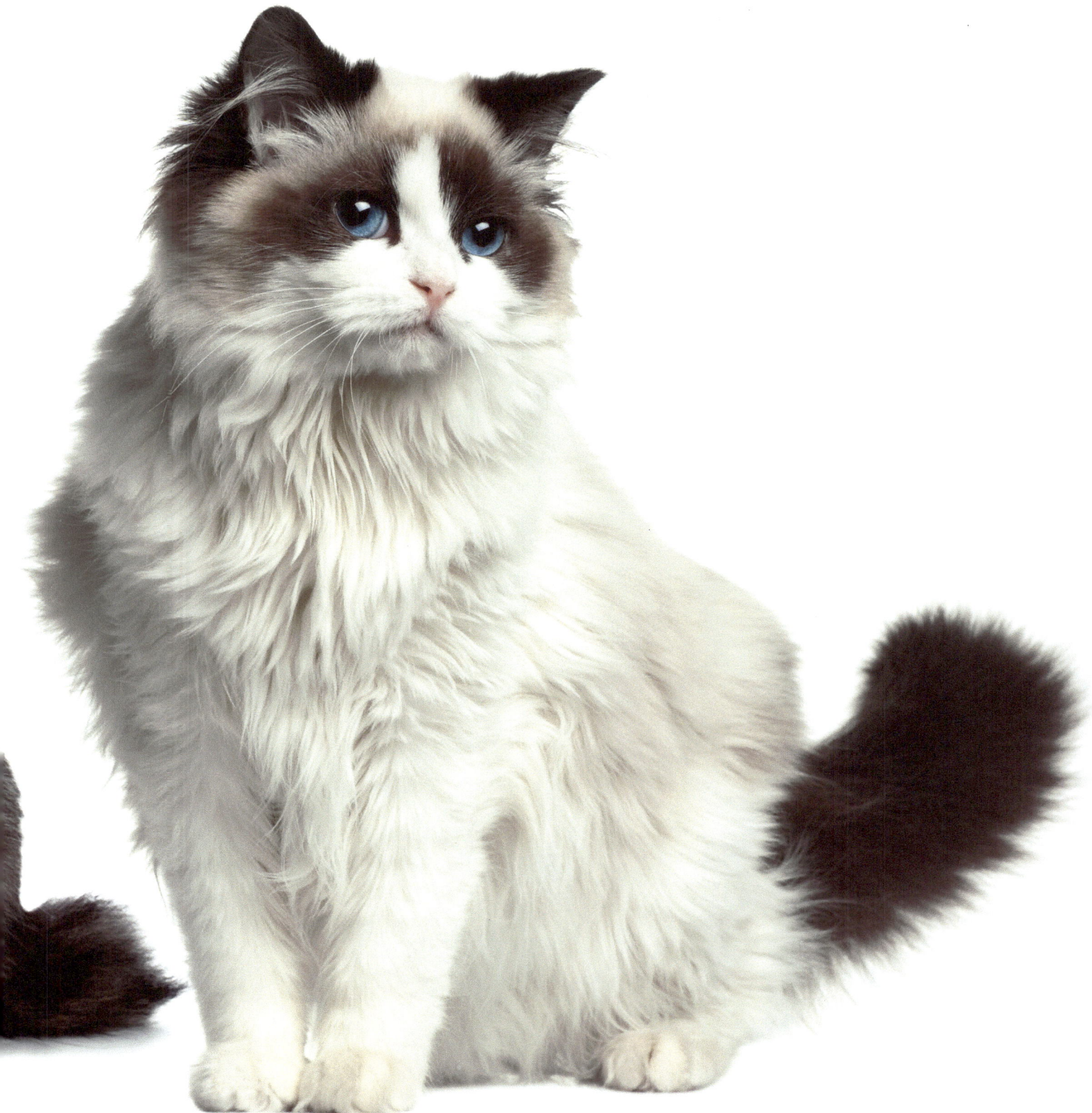

Ragdoll

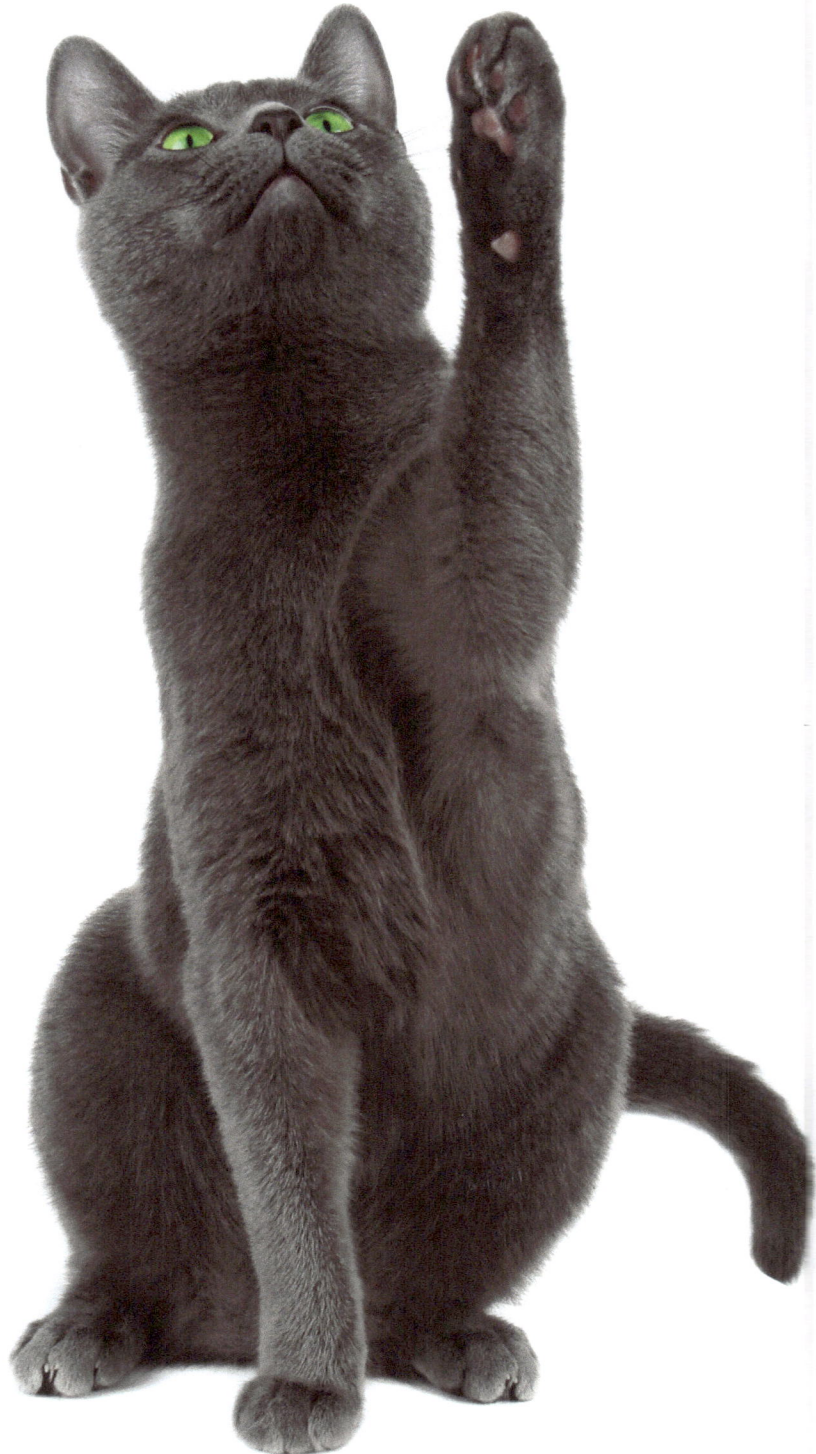

Russian Blue

Savannah

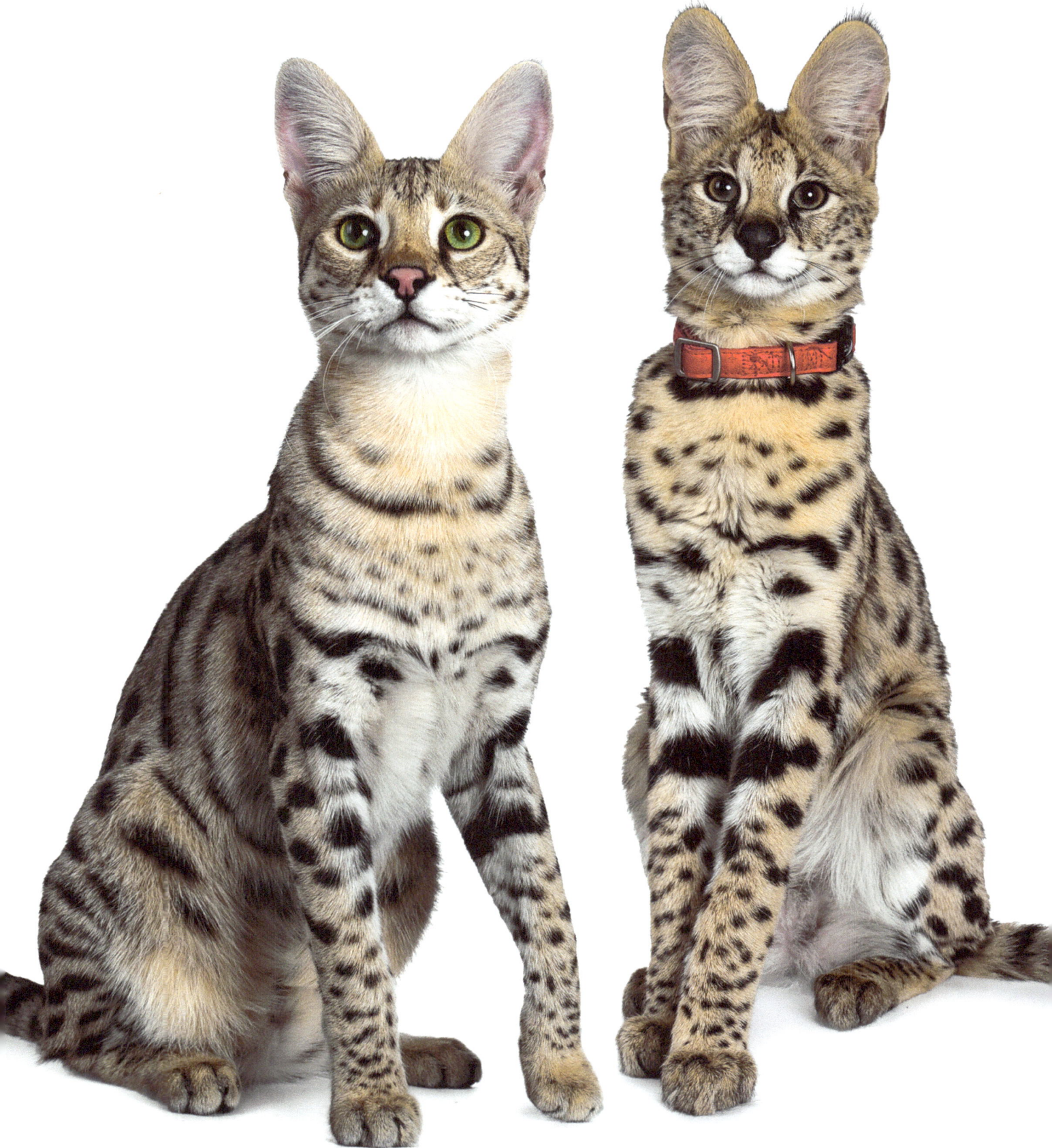

Scottish Fold

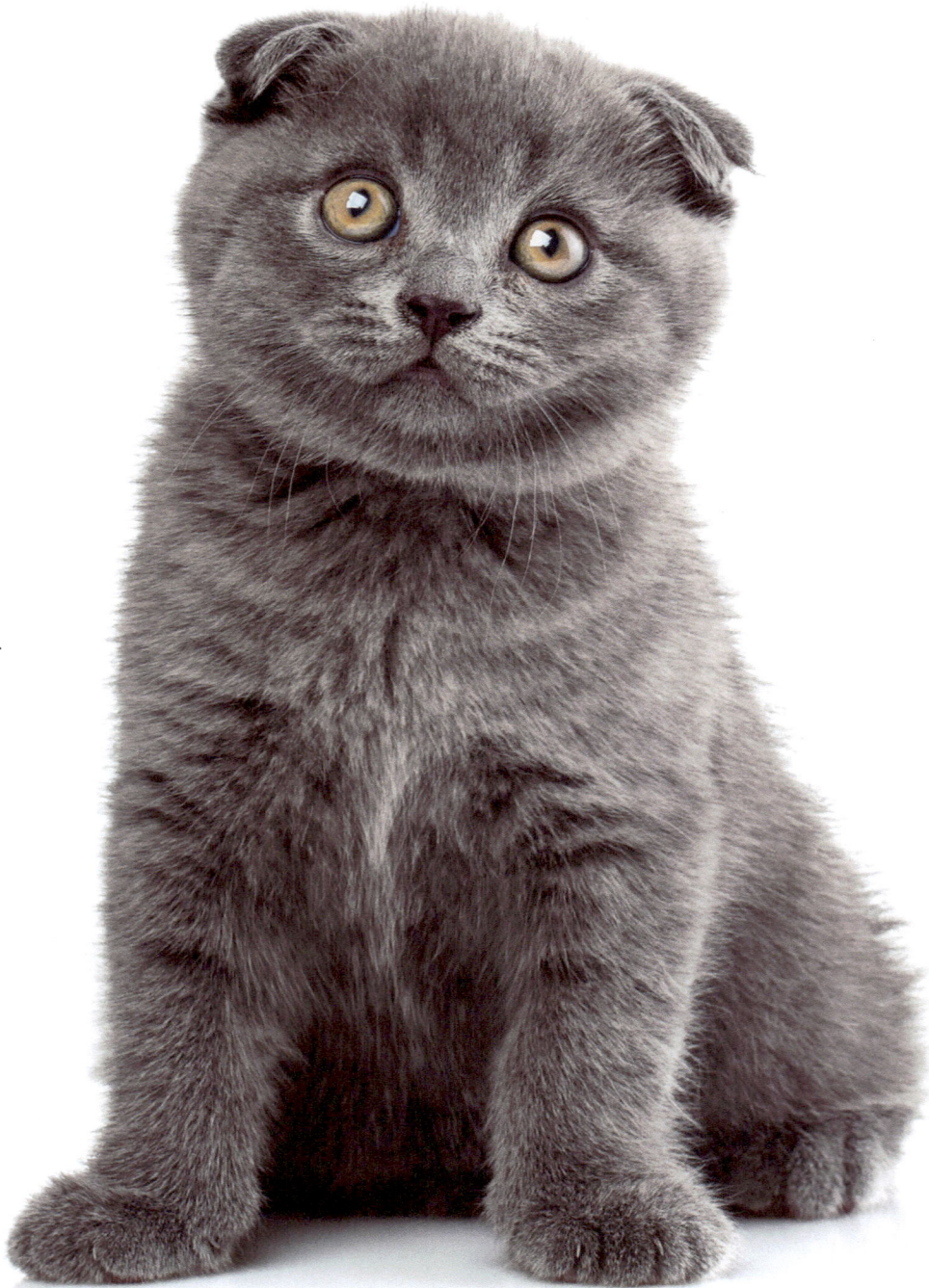

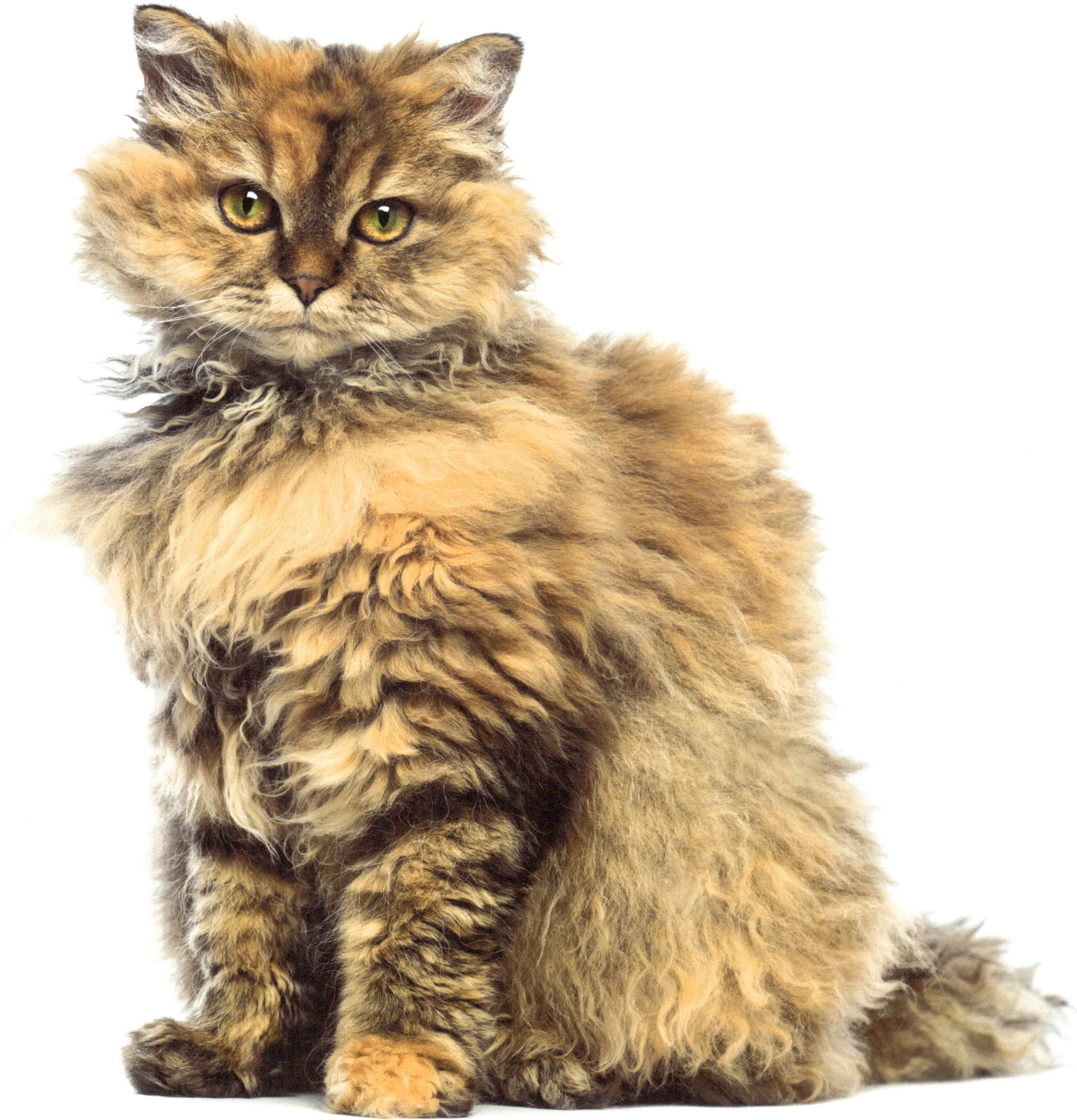

Selkirk Rex

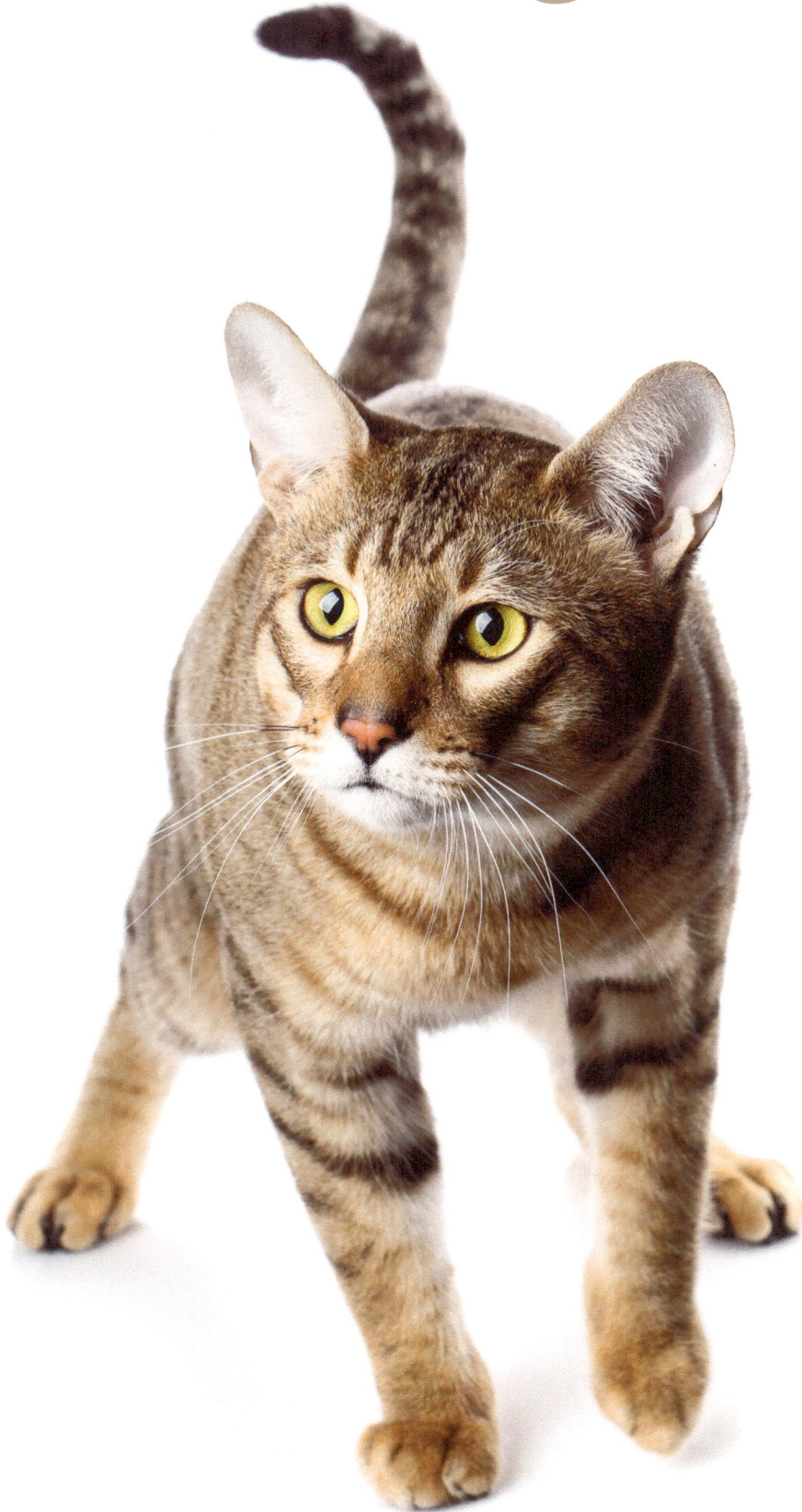

Serengeti

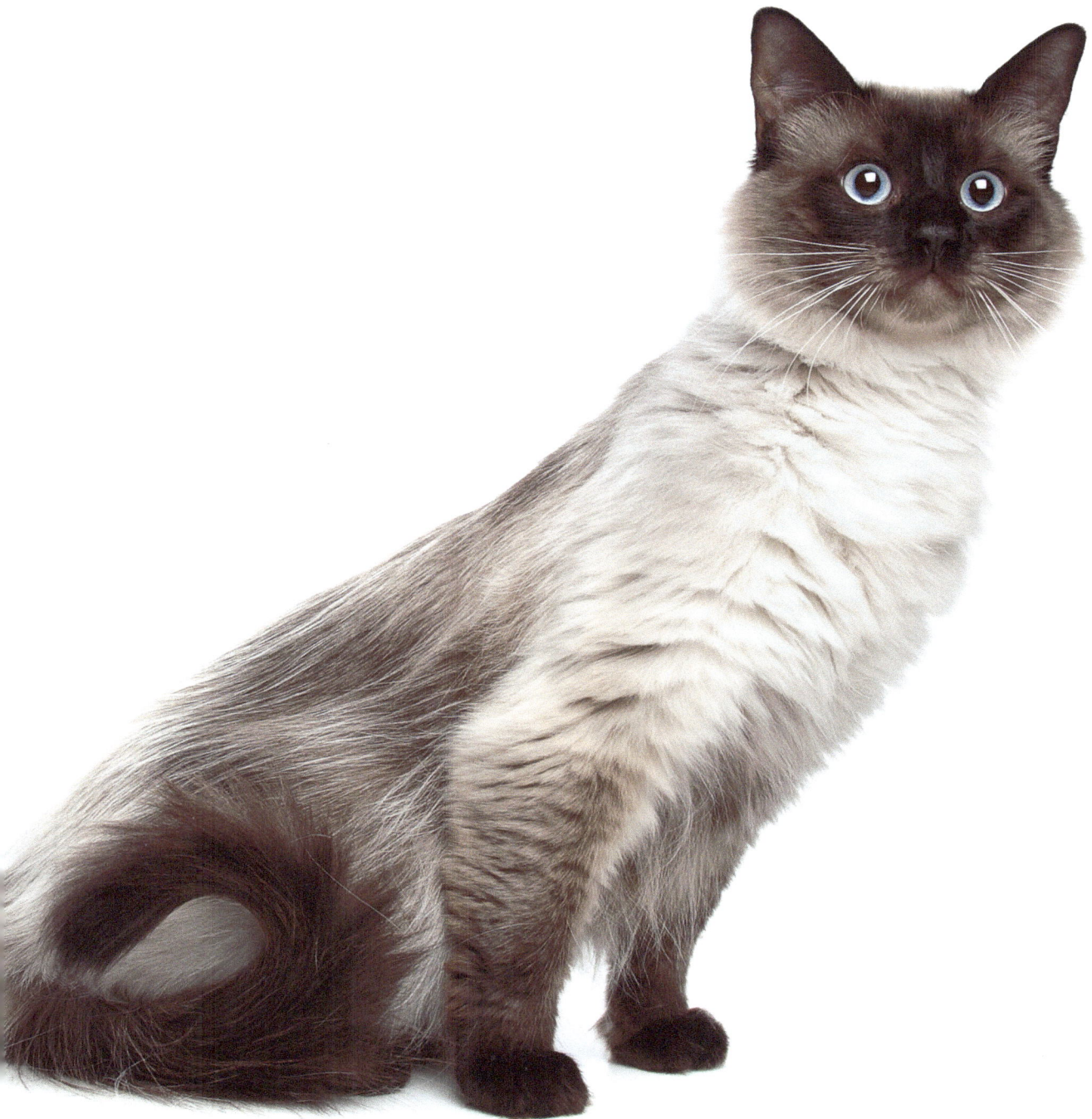

Siamese

Siberian Forest

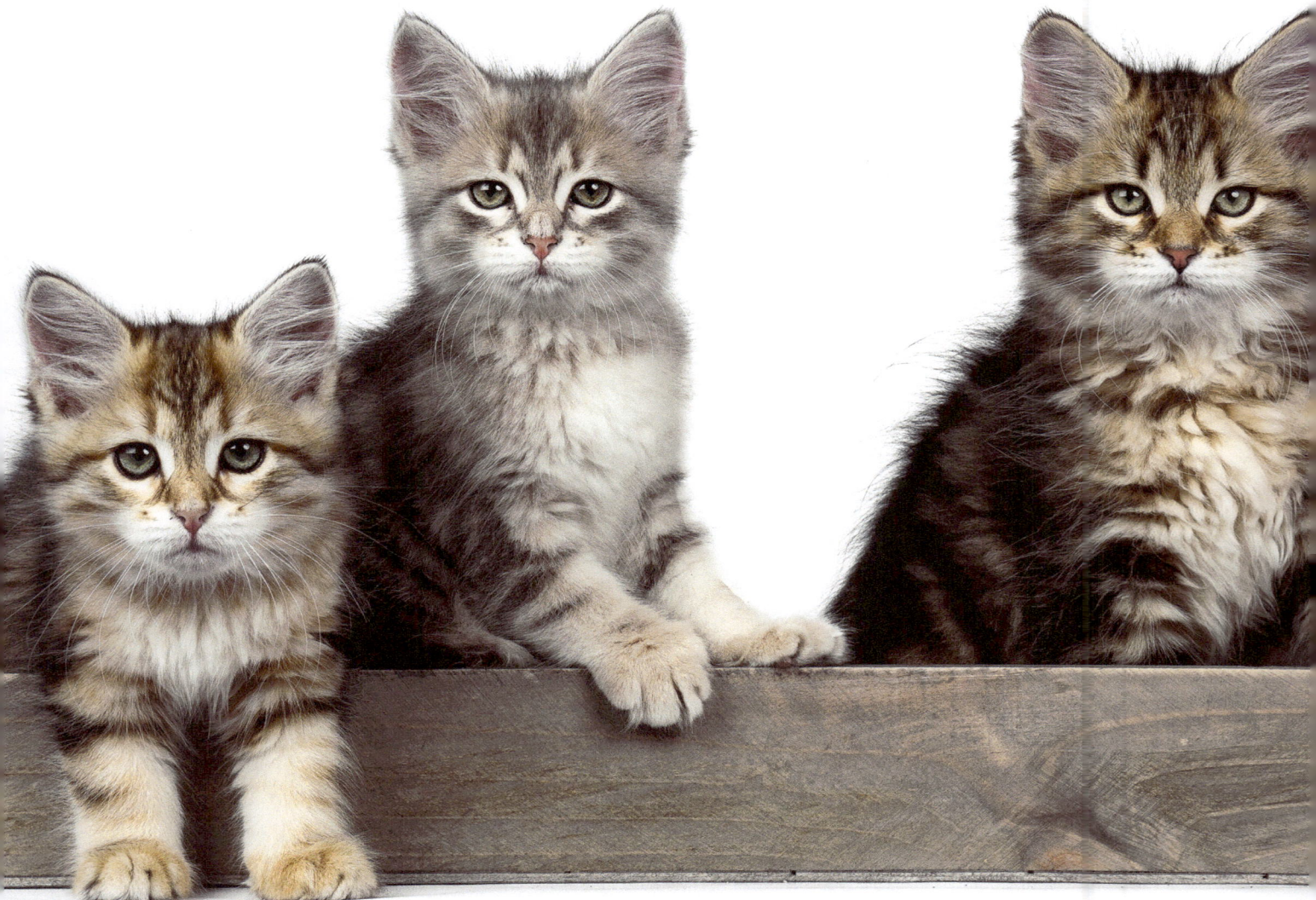

Singapura

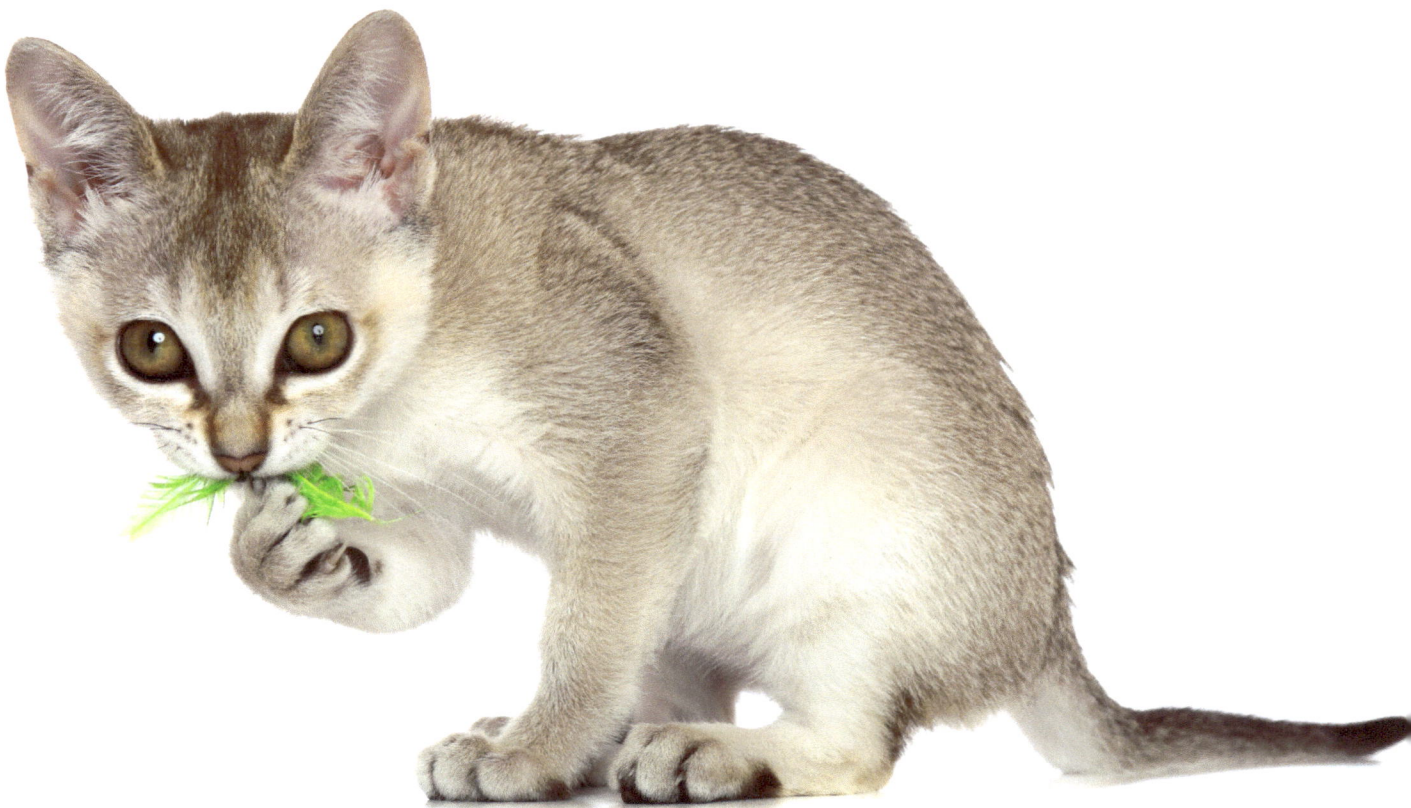

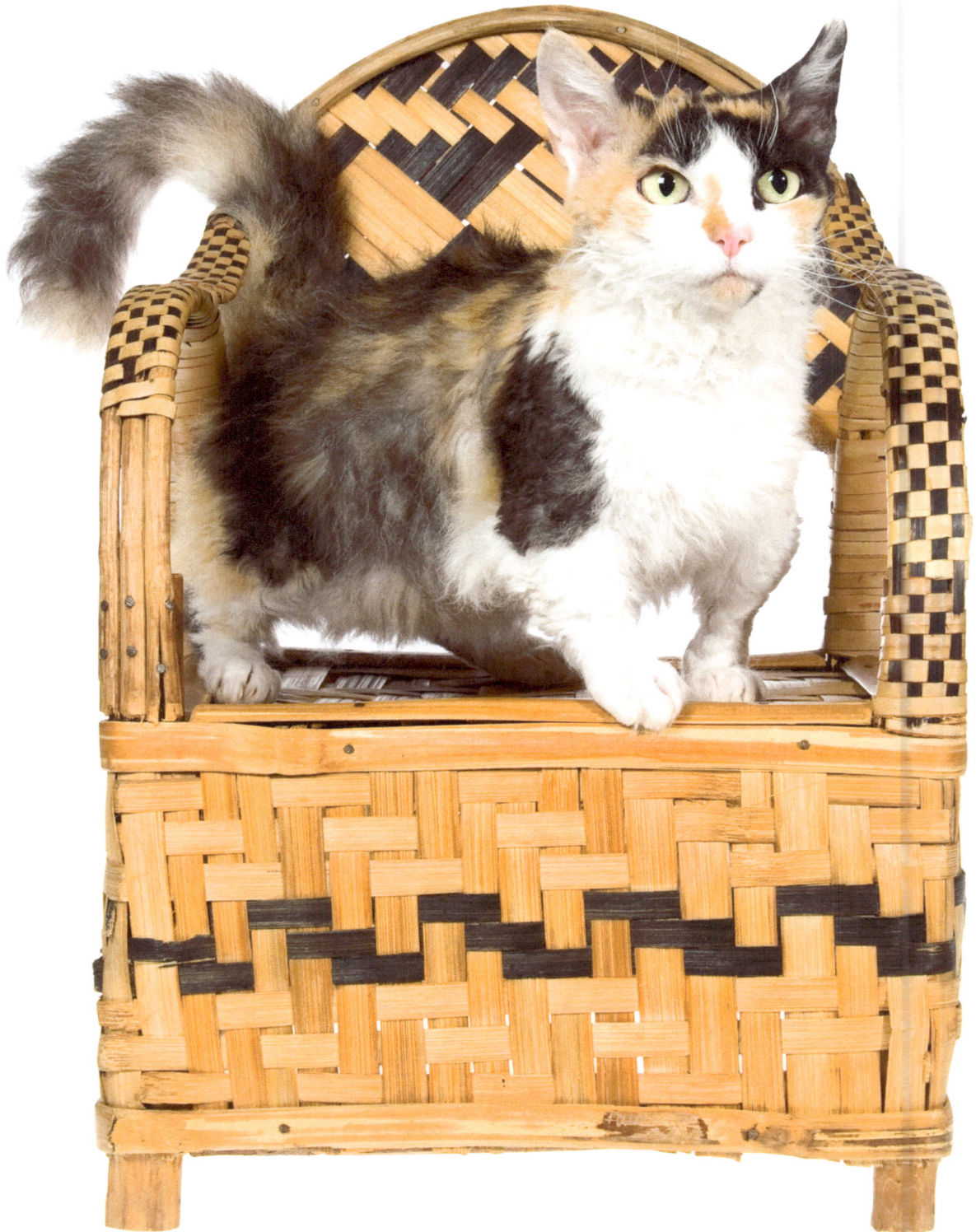

Skookum

Snowshoe

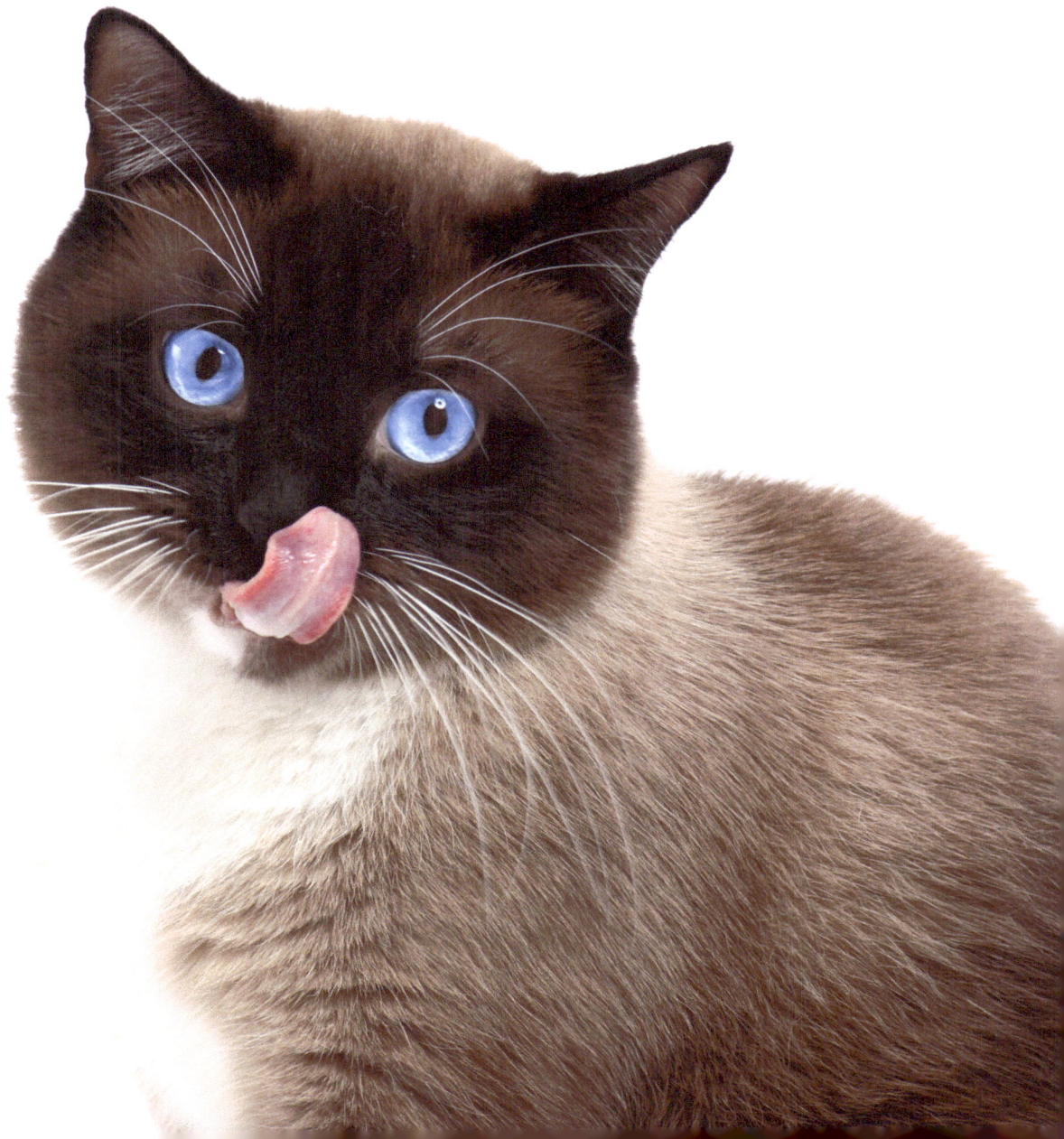

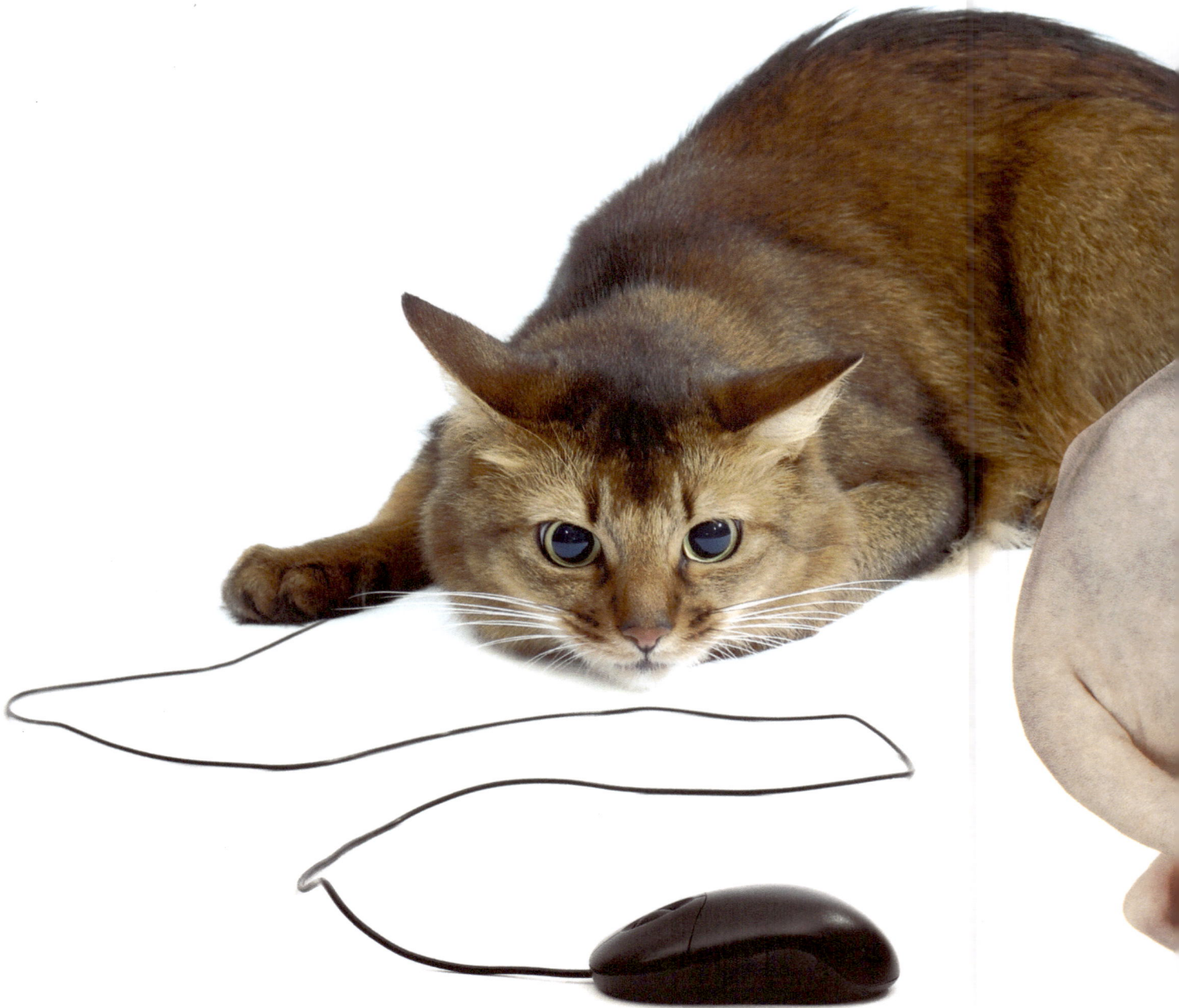

Somali

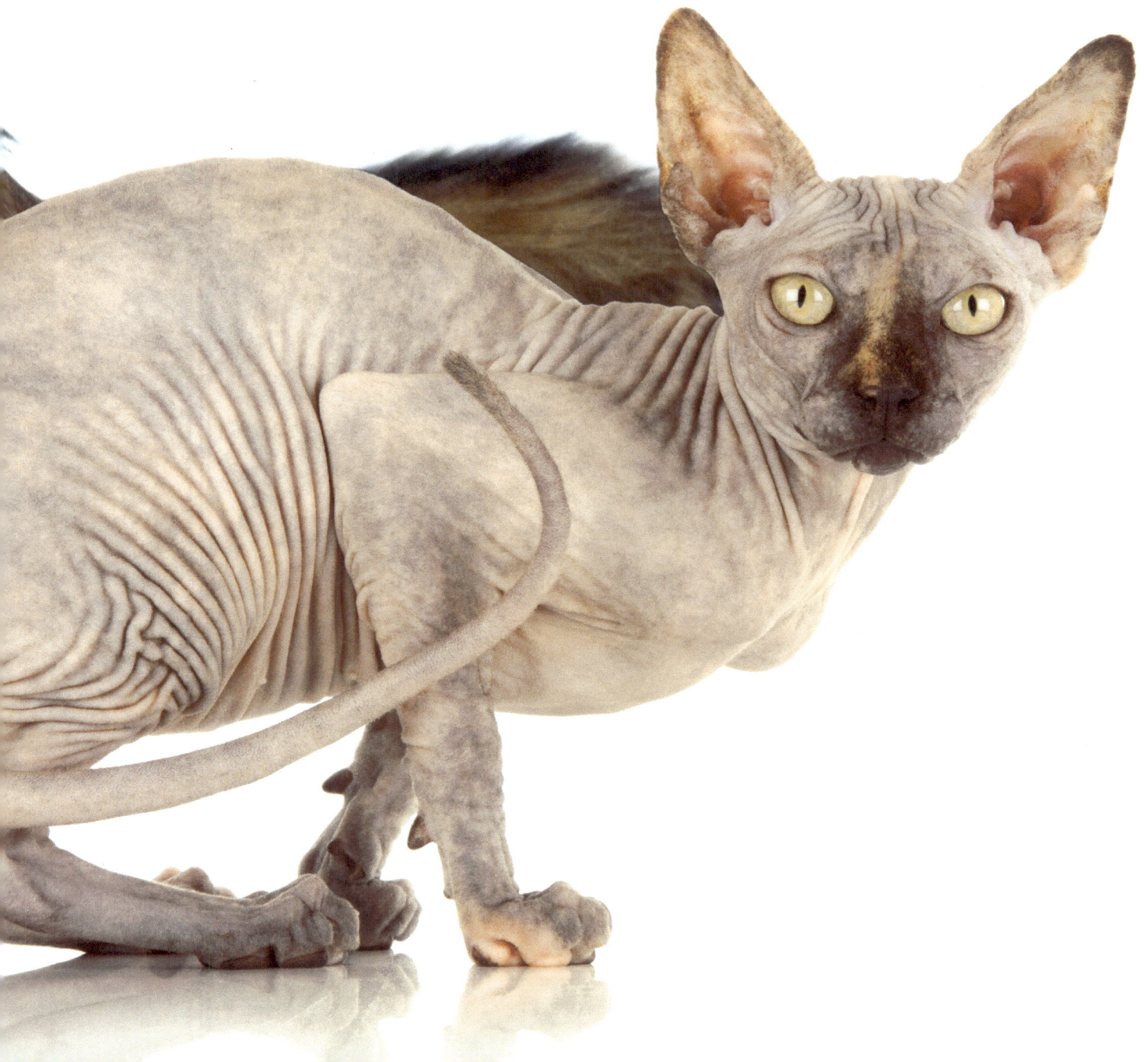

Sphynx

Tonkinese

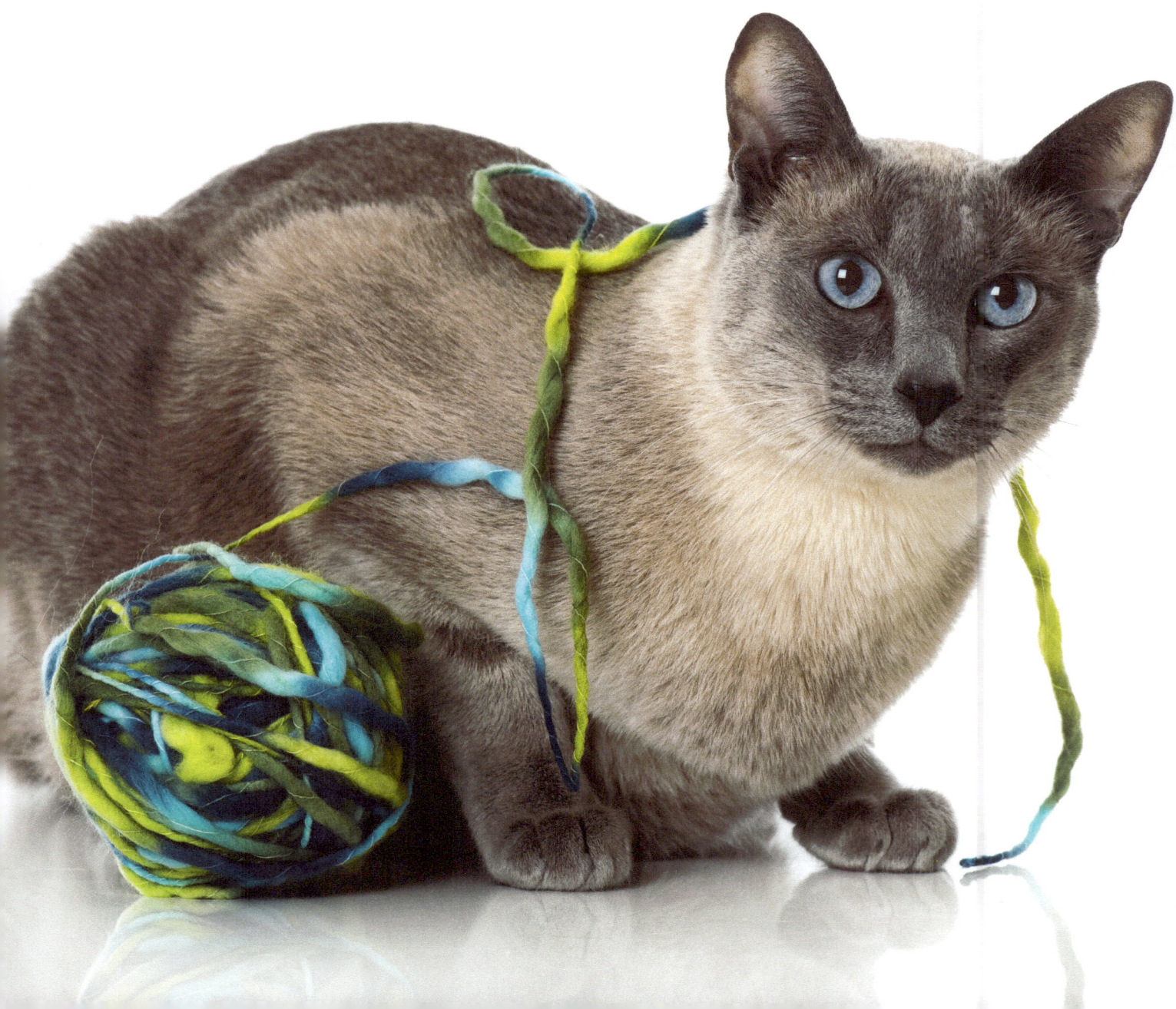

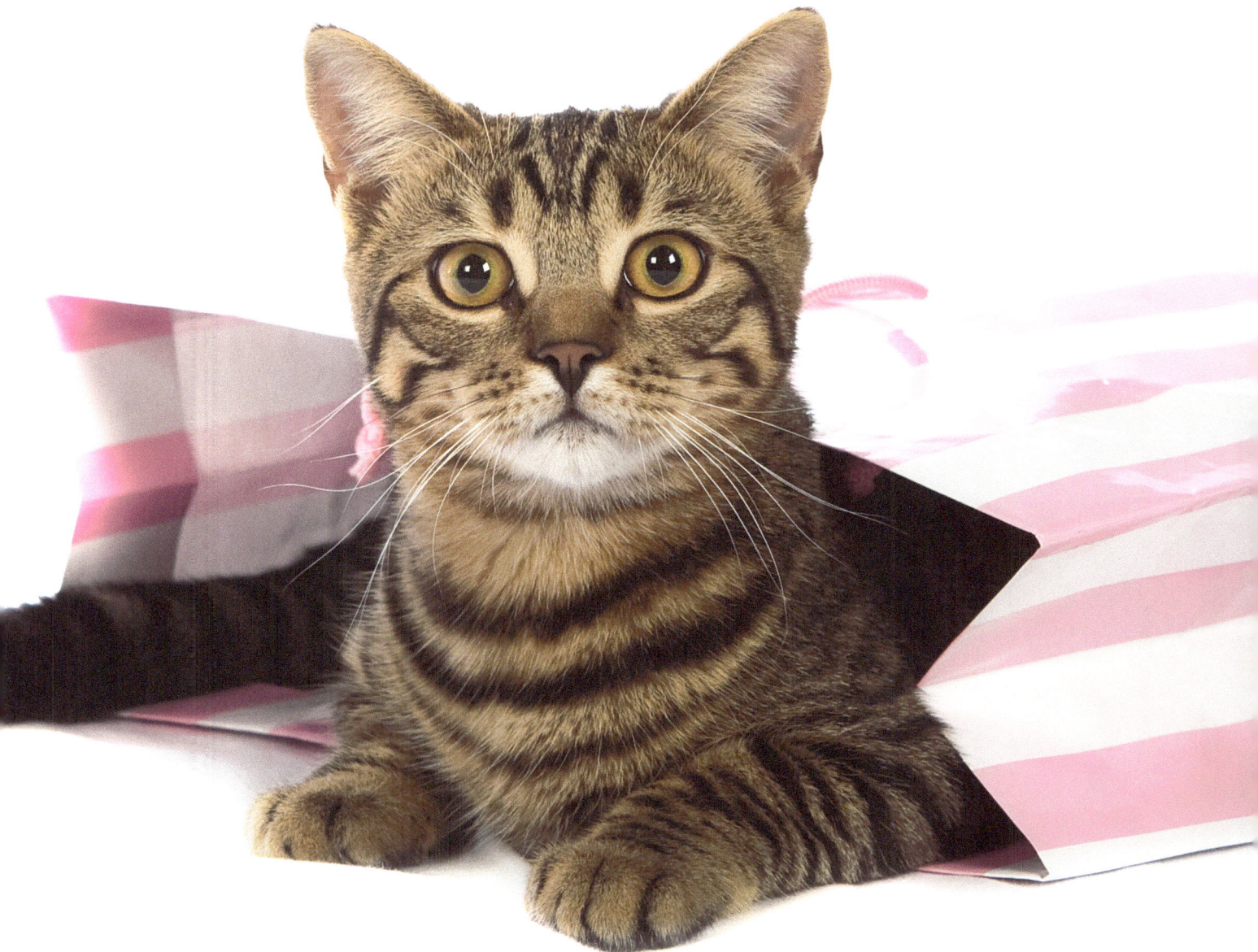

Toyger

Turkish Angora

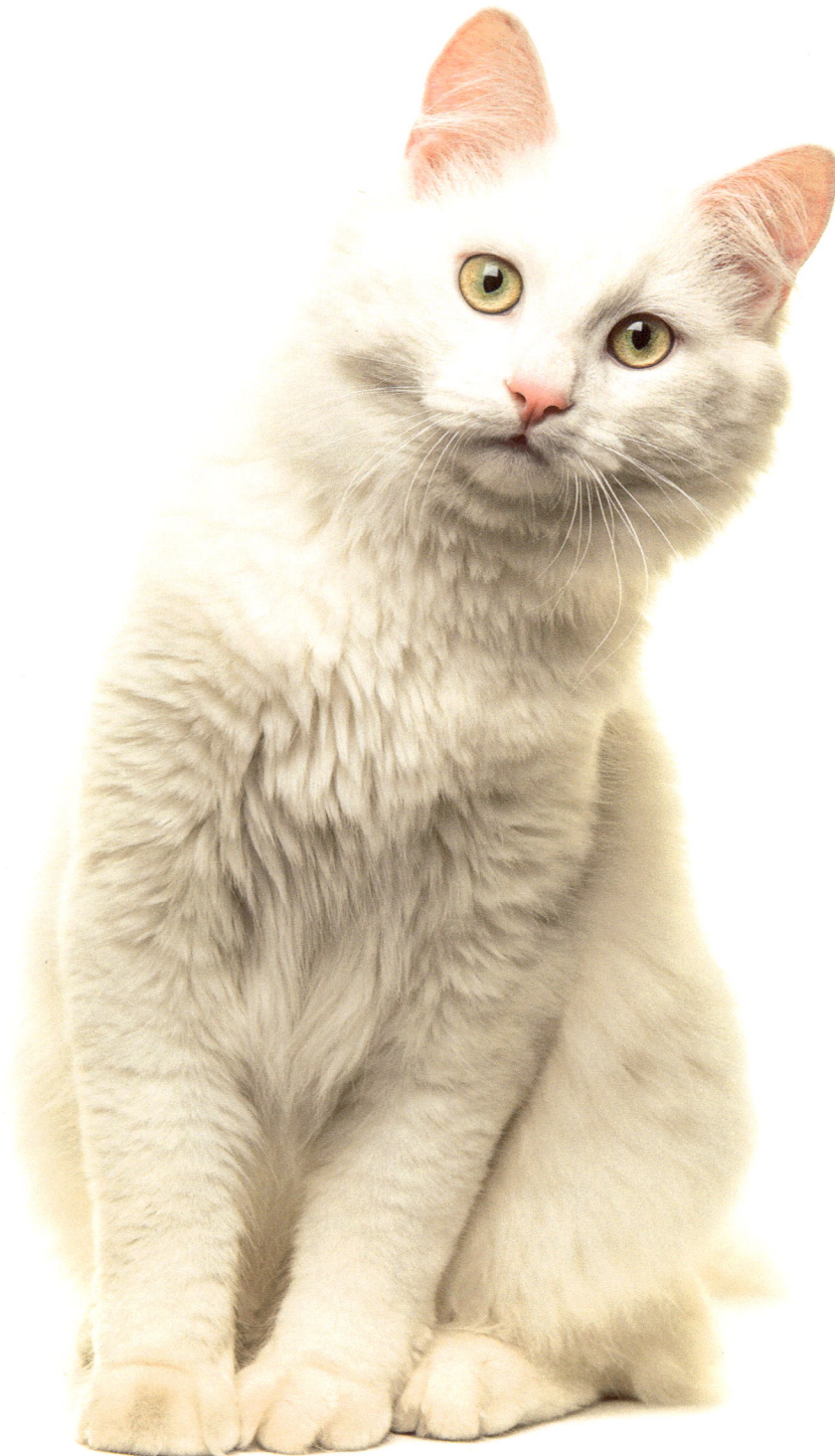

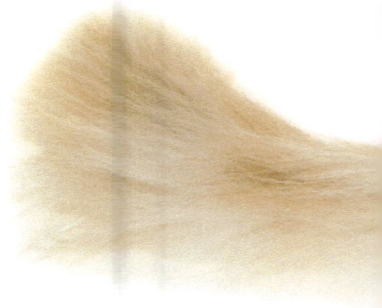

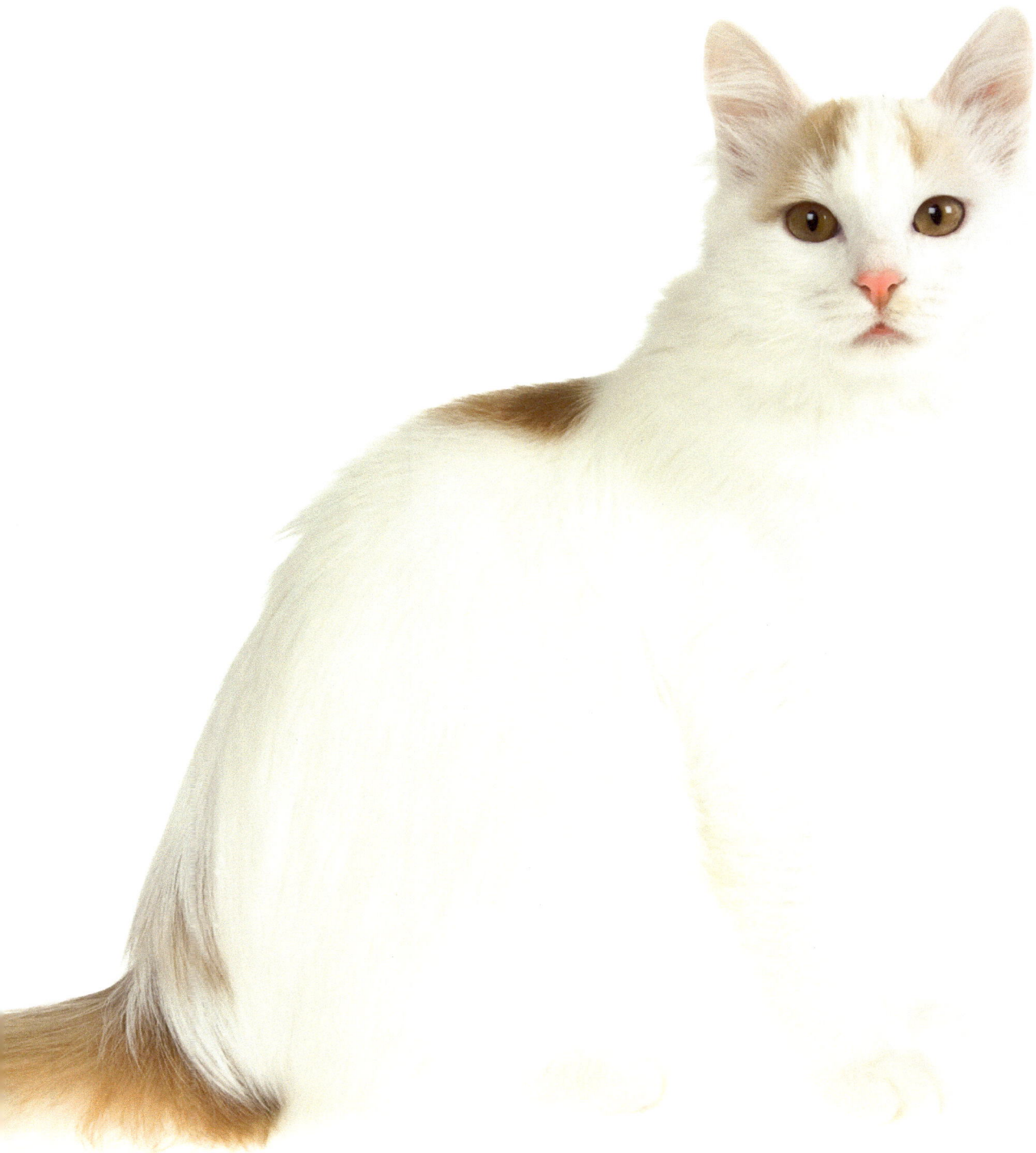

Turkish Van

www.ingramcontent.com/pod-product-compliance
Lightning Source LLC
Chambersburg PA
CBHW041544260326

41914CB00015B/1542